Cautious Care: A Guide for Patients

Don't assume your medical care is "good enough."

Cautious Care: A Guide for Patients

⌖

What you don't know may harm you.

Carolyn Oliver, M.D., J.D.

Cautious Care: A Guide for Patients
by Carolyn Oliver

January, 2009
USA

1. Health. 2. Medical care. 3. Patient safety. 4. Medical errors.
5. Patient advocacy. 6. Patient empowerment.
7. Misdiagnosed.

Order from Amazon.com

Coliver.MD@gmail.com

This book is meant to help you get safe, effective, less frustrating medical care; but please see a physician anytime you feel you have a medical situation. The intent of the author of this book is only to offer information of a general nature.

ISBN: 1440418675

EAN 13: 978-1440418679

"Each year, 100,000 Americans die because of medical errors ..."

Senator Barack Obama

Obama, Barack. "Affordable Health Care for All Americans: The Obama-Biden Plan."*Journal of the American Medical Association* 300(16) (2008): 1927-1928.

"I understand that when Medicare squeezes providers to lower the cost of care, the result is distortion of the care that patients receive ..."

Senator John McCain

McCain, John. "Access to Quality and Affordable Health Care for Every American." *New England Journal of Medicine* 359(15) (2008): 1537-1541.

"We all know the statistic from the landmark 1999 Institute of Medicine report that as many as 98,000 deaths in the United States each year result from medical errors."

Hillary Rodham Clinton and Barack Obama

Clinton, Hillary Rodham and Barack Obama. "Making Patient Safety the Centerpiece of Medical Liability Reform." *New England Journal of Medicine* 354(21) (2006): 2205-2208.

Table of Contents

Instructions for Using This Guide

Please Read This

This guide is meant to be used *either* by the patient himself *or* by a loved one who is watching out for a patient, like a parent, spouse/mate, or other loved one.

As such, the Guide is sometimes in the form of advice given to the loved one and sometimes in advice to the patient himself. In either case, the patient or loved one will easily see what needs to be done. Use this advice to get the respect, consideration, and satisfaction that we all should get from the healthcare system, but that has become sorely lacking.

The Guide is meant to be, and is, an easy read. Your role in getting what you need from your healthcare encounters will be best understood by reading straight through the book and not just picking topics. Then read the Endnotes *after* the body of the book. You'll understand them better at the end, and they'll add and give substance to what you've learned in the core of the book.

Once you've read Chapter One, you cannot go back to being uninformed. Once you see the danger, you must do what you can for your loved one.

Here's hoping that you will be brave enough to respectfully but firmly insist on your right to take care of yourself or your loved one. The healthcare system will not change until most of us respectfully but firmly assert our right—*and* accept our responsibility—to help.

Chapter One

If You Believe ...

If you believe that

doctors are fallible*

*fallible – capable of making an error
(American Heritage Dictionary, Fourth Edition)

If you believe that

you have more interest and investment in the welfare of your loved one than the doctor does

If you believe that

you have more time to think about what is best for your loved one than a doctor has

If you believe that

you know your loved one better than a doctor ever could

If you believe that

most doctors no longer have the time to do the "best" job for their patients

If you believe that

many doctors are controlling and arrogant (and some wield their power over you in an insensitive fashion)

If you believe that

doctors are human, and come with all the usual human foibles, such as pride and greed

If you believe that

doctors and nurses are human, and can't make good decisions in a sleep-deprived state any better than you could, or than an airline pilot could

If you believe that

doctors are human, and as such, have about the same rates of alcohol abuse, drug abuse and personality disorders as the rest of the people in the United States

If you believe that

doctors are subject to the same everyday troubles that weigh on their minds and can distract them from their jobs (you!) as everybody else in the work force (problems with finances, marriages, teenagers, illnesses, time constraints)

If you believe that

nurses and other medical personnel have these same distractions, and because of this, at any time could make an error that could change your life forever

If you believe that

some doctors, despite their charms, professional appearances or qualifications, are actually looking out *first* for their bottom lines (profits), and only *secondarily* at your best interests, and that you can't really tell the difference between them and the "good" doctors—that is, there are some doctors who are "operators" and it's nearly impossible to spot them

If you believe that

like priests, doctors are in an important, authoritarian position to influence our lives profoundly—either for the good or the bad

If you believe that

the state medical boards that license and police our doctors have low budgets and little power, and so can only deal with the doctors who are the most flagrant in their abuses against the public; thus, each physician has somewhat a little kingdom of his own

If you believe that

"absolute power corrupts absolutely"*

*Attributed to John Emerich Edward Dalberg Acton, first Baron Acton (1834-1902)

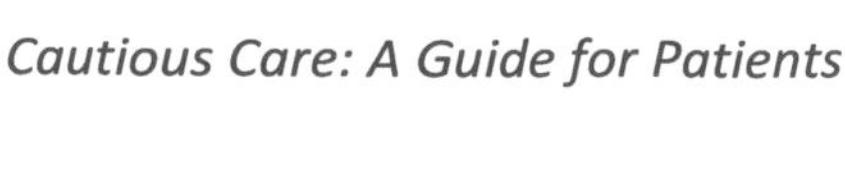

If you believe that

some auto mechanics or repairmen may tell you something is wrong, so that they can get paid to “fix it” (and you understand that some doctors have the same base instincts)

If you believe that

many doctors and nurses are doing the right thing—but that there are still some things that you should know to help them help you

If you believe that

even more doctors and nurses are *trying* to do the right thing, but can't keep up with the ever-increasing list of bureaucratic demands that our current, dysfunctional healthcare system places on them

If you believe that

many doctors have to work in situations where they are told how many patients they need to see per day, even though they feel like that is not enough time to do right by the patient

If you believe that

many hospital nurses are told by hospital administrators how many patients they have to take care of, and even though the nurses *know* it's an unreasonable request, there's no way for them to protect patients from what they believe to be unsafe staffing

If you believe that

some doctors, nurses and other medical personnel get "hardened" to the suffering and pain of others, not because they want to be, but because they somewhat have to be in order to do what they do; and that often a patient's family can help prevent some suffering by *being there* to remind the doctor or nurse to be gentler with the patient

If you believe that

as many people *die* from *medical errors* in U.S. hospitals each year as would occur if a commercial jet crashed *each day of the year* (almost 100,000 lives per year)[1]; and that number doesn't include the thousands who survive medical mistakes but suffer unnecessarily or become permanently disabled; and that number doesn't include the 99,000 people who die each year from infections acquired in the hospital; and that number doesn't include those who die or are permanently harmed while being treated *outside* of the hospital

[1] – More info on this topic in Endnote 1 at the back of the book.

If you believe that

we don't hear about many of the people who've died or are disabled due to medical errors because our legal system allows the doctor and his attorney to require the injured patient or patient's family to sign a non-disclosure clause (more or less, a gag order) to settle the case

If you believe that

other reasons that we don't *get it* that we need to take steps to try to protect ourselves from fatal medical errors are that the numbers trickle in across the country daily in non-sensational ways[2] (unlike airplane crashes), and we wrongly believe that these errors only occur occasionally, sensationally to "bad doctors" like the ones we've seen on TV news programs

If you believe that

many people in the U.S. with chronic health problems, like diabetes, high blood pressure, asthma and heart disease, aren't given the medical advice and medical management recommended by prominent medical authorities, that could help them live healthier, happier, and longer lives[3]

If you believe that

many patients and families are suffering today because of mis-managed, undiagnosed or misdiagnosed health problems[4]

If you believe that

you are in a safe spot with "your doctor" (but you're taking that completely on hope and faith, and aren't taking the steps along the way to double-check)

If you believe that

hiding your head in the sand to the facts would be wrong

If you believe that

it would be wrong for you to know all these facts to be true, and yet with blind faith hand over the complete medical care of your loved one to our flawed healthcare system

If you believe that

if your loved one was injured or died because of medical error, then *you* could have been one of the people who might have prevented it

If you believe *any* of these things to be true

then you must take action to ensure the safety and well-being of your loved one.

Chapter Two

Your Responsibility

or

With Knowledge Comes Responsibility

I know the statements in the previous chapter to be true.

If you don't have the time, or have the time and don't make the effort, to do *the best you can* to protect yourself or your loved one in the healthcare system, then *you* could be one of the hundreds of thousands of Americans every year who rolls the dice and takes his chances, but *loses* in this deadly game, resulting in death or permanent disability because of a medical error.[1]

Or you might be one of those with a chronic disease who is only partially treated, and so you unnecessarily develop complications (blindness, kidney disease, heart attacks) or die earlier than you needed to—both of which could have been prevented with proper treatment.[3]

Because, if the healthcare system is broken (which it is), and there are things that you can do to help (which there are), how can you ignore your responsibility?

Chapter Three

Your Responsibility as an Outpatient

"In sum, health care is plagued today by a serious quality gap."*

*Institute of Medicine. *Crossing the Quality Chasm: A New Health System for the 21st Century*. Washington, D.C.: National Academy Press, 2001, p. 35.

Basically, there are two separate medical scenarios: being an "outpatient"—being treated by a doctor when *not* in a hospital, and being an "inpatient"—being treated by a doctor while *in* a hospital.

This chapter is advice to use when you are an outpatient.

Your number one most important asset for getting good medical care

• You need to make and keep a "personal health record."

Because of time constraints, doctors in our medical system often treat you *without enough information about you*, with devastating results. Don't just take my word for it. See Appendix A for further documenting information.

Here are the real facts about medical care today: Doctors see twenty or more patients daily. Each patient's medical chart is a pile of papers that the doctor doesn't have time to go through and organize properly. Doctors who properly keep a patient's medical information in the form of a current problem list, a current medication list, and an easily-accessible history about your diseases, hospitalizations, lab tests, and procedures, have disappeared with the advent of managed care, cost-cutting, patients changing doctors frequently due to changes in their jobs or healthcare benefits, and drugstore clinics.

And even if *your* doctor is one of the few that keeps that record truly organized, if you're seeing more than one doctor, it's almost certain that you don't have a *complete* record of your health information anywhere.

So, the simplest, most pro-active and important thing you can do to keep yourself safe in healthcare is to keep your own medical record—what is called a "personal health record."

But don't just go typing a list of your medicines, or saving a stack of your lab results, because doctors will *almost never* have the time or incentive to look at those things, because they're not organized in the format that doctors like to use to look at records.

Doctors like to see medical information organized in a certain format, and the best thing you can do to help yourself get the best medical care and avoid dangerous care is to put your medical information into that form, and to keep it updated. Then print it out and take it with you whenever you see a doctor.

You can't put this off until later or "whenever"—do it now. We'll show you how to do that in Appendix B.

And don't make the mistake of thinking "I'm really healthy—I just don't need to do that, because I don't have any problems."

Here's the problem with that: you may not have any medical problems, but unless you give the doctor your personal health record that lets him see your "I'm healthy" history in an organized way, then a good doctor still has to take the time *to ask you* a long list of questions about your health, and then organize that information, instead of spending his time (and your time) focusing on the problem at hand and getting straight to a proper diagnosis and treatment.

Many of you, when you first read this piece of advice, will say, "Yeah—no. I'm too busy, and I just don't want to go to all that trouble."

Keep reading this book, and by the time you get to the end, I'm thinking you'll see things differently.

> "The meticulous collection of personal health information throughout a patient's life can be one of the most important inputs to the provision of proper care. Yet for most individuals, that health information is dispersed in a collection of paper records that are poorly organized and often illegible, and frequently cannot be retrieved in a timely fashion, making it nearly impossible to manage many forms of chronic illness that require frequent monitoring and ongoing patient support."*

It will only take 20-30 minutes. See Appendices A and B on how to proceed.

*Institute of Medicine. *Crossing the Quality Chasm: A New Health System for the 21st Century*. Washington, D.C.: National Academy Press, 2001, p. 15.

Remember when your doctor used to talk to you? – Thank goodness you now have other options

• Many of us can remember a time twenty years or so ago when doctors seemed kind and spent time talking to us and listening to us. That was not only good bedside manners—that was *good medicine.* A doctor can't really tell what's wrong with a patient unless he *listens* to him, and a doctor can't really treat the patient well unless he *answers* the patient's questions.

But those days are mostly over.

Now the pace of medicine is frantic, and studies show that, on average, a patient talks for less than 30 seconds before the doctor interrupts him.

Medicine has changed, and not for the better.

Doctors don't like it, nurses don't like it, and patients don't like it. And it won't get better until there are *big* changes in the bureaucratic pressures under which most doctors and nurses work today.

But not to despair—doctors no longer hold the keys to all things medical. Support for you has arrived, literally at your fingertips—the computer and the Internet.

If you access reputable medical websites for information on your illnesses, you can learn so much more than what your doctor has the time to tell you.

And what you learn can be lifesaving.

And, sometimes, what you can learn and find out about your health on the Internet *is better* than what your doctor can tell you. You'll learn more about this later.

Of course, the best of all worlds would be an up-to-date, organized, rested, unhurried, honest, kind and sympathetic doctor who has the time to tell you everything you need to know when you go to him for his advice on how to gain and maintain good health.

Let's work toward that goal—but in the meantime, let's make sure that your health is taken care of when your medical care falls short of that vision. Keep reading for lots of ways to do this.

"The specter of a 7-minute doctor office visit, during which government-imposed checklists and managed care clinical pathways must be addressed, is not a welcome development for many physicians."*

"When you do get an appointment, you wait an excessive time before seeing the doctor, who is in a hurry, does not seem to care, and provides inadequate explanation and education."†

*Beck, Arne, John Scott, and Patrick Williams et al. "A Randomized Trial of Group Outpatient Visits for Chronically Ill Older HMO Members: The Cooperative Health Care Clinic." *Journal of the American Geriatrics Society* 45(5) (1997): 543-549.

†Kuzel, Anton J., Steven H. Woolf, and Valerie J. Gilchrist et al. "Patient Reports of Preventable Problems and Harms in Primary Heath Care." *Annals of Family Medicine* 2 (2004): 333-340. This quote summarized how many patients in the survey felt about their current healthcare situation.

A real Catch-22 (and what you don't know can hurt you)

The amount of *time* your doctor *is able* to spend with you

has not kept pace

with the amount of time *it would take him*

to tell you all of the things that he now knows

can help you live your longest, healthiest life!

• SO, if you are one of the 100 million Americans with one or more chronic diseases like diabetes, high blood pressure, asthma, high cholesterol or heart disease, we now have evidence-based medicine that recommends almost exactly how you should be treated to get the best results—longer, healthier lives with less complications—but your doctor doesn't have the time to spend with you to get you to the point of best results![*, †]

THUS, over 4 out of every 10 patients with a chronic illness get only *partially* treated, so they cannot expect to live their longest, healthiest lives just from the advice their doctor has the time to tell them.[3]

AND, we now know about the value of *preventive medicine interventions*—about vaccines, pap smears, mammograms, colonoscopies, blood pressure checks, cholesterol checks and so on—so that you can live your longest, healthiest life—but your doctor doesn't have the time to tell you what you need and to guide you to get it done![*, †]

THUS, over 4 out of every 10 patients get only *partial* advice on prevention, so—well, you get the picture.[3]

For most of the centuries in the history of medicine, doctors had very few tricks in their bags. Medicine was usually about common-sense folk remedies, splinting bones, rudimentary surgery, comforting patients, and decreasing suffering.

Before the 1940s, we had only a handful of useful medications, such as digitalis, morphine, and sulfa.

Then medical knowledge started steamrolling along with the rest of scientific knowledge. By the 1970s, about 100 new reliable medical studies were done each year that could give meaningful information to doctors on how to cure some diseases and control others. Today, there are 10,000 of those studies published every year.

And wouldn't you know it—now that we have so much more really accurate medical knowledge about the intricacies of diseases, preventive medicine and medications to keep you from dying early and keep you well for a long time without complications from your chronic diseases—doctors are given less and less time to spend with their patients, due to managed care, government demands and bureaucratic pressures.

A perfect Catch-22—so much knowledge to impart, so little time.

The only thing that I can suggest to you is that *you* take the initiative to find out what you need to do to live your longest and healthiest life with your chronic illness. *You* take the initiative to find out what preventive tests you should be taking to give yourself the best chance at living your longest and healthiest life.

Only you can do it.

But you have help. The Cautious Patient organization at www.CautiousPatient.org will help you find all of the information your doctor doesn't have the time to tell you about your chronic diseases or preventive medicine.

And by the way—if you already have your medical information in a personal health record that is in an organized, printed form that doctors like to use—then your doctor will need to spend less time quizzing you about your medical history, and more time being able to treat you and tell you things you should know. So don't even try to get the *best* medical care without it. See more in Appendices A and B.

"There is a sharp, persistent divide between health professionals' *knowledge* of what constitutes best practices and the care that is *actually delivered*."*

"The time needed to meet preventive, chronic, and acute care requirements *vastly exceeds the total time physicians have available* for patient care … Americans receive *only about one half* of the applicable services for acute, preventive, and chronic disease care … The human costs are substantial: poor blood pressure control contributes to *more than 68,000 preventable deaths annually*, and strict blood glucose control can decrease the risk of complications in patients with diabetes by 25%."†

"Health care today is characterized by more to know, more to manage, more to watch, more to do, and more people involved in doing it than at any time in the nation's history. Our current methods of organizing and delivering care are unable to meet the expectations of patients and their families because *the science technologies involved in health care*—the knowledge, skills, care interventions, devices, and drugs—*have advanced more rapidly than our ability to deliver them safely, effectively, and efficiently*."‡

*Blumenthal, David, and Charles M. Kilo. "A Report Card on Continuous Quality Improvement." *The Milbank Quarterly* 76(4) (1998): 625-648, *italics added.*

†Ostbye, Truls, Kimberly S.H. Yarnall, Katrina M. Krause, Kathryn I. Pollak, Margaret Gradison, and J. Lloyd Michener. "Is There Time for Management of Patients with Chronic Diseases in Primary care? *Annals of Family Medicine* 3(3) (2005): 209-214, *italics added.*

‡Institute of Medicine. *Crossing the Quality Chasm: A New Health System for the 21st Century*. Washington, D.C.: National Academy Press, 2001, p. 25, *italics added.*

First obstacle to get past in the doctor's office

• Be cautious in a doctor's office that has the nurse interview you at the beginning of your office visit, and she writes some things down for the doctor before the doctor comes in. Chances are she will not write down everything you tell her, and she may not use *your own words*—both of which may be important for your correct diagnosis.

Some doctors do this because an x-ray or lab test can be ordered right away, and would need to be done before the doctor makes a diagnosis, and that makes sense. Also, if you have a pretty simple problem like just a sore throat, there may not be any harm in this approach.

But other times, it can be a "shortcut" for a doctor who really should be hearing all of your symptoms himself, but he thinks this is a time-saver. When that is the case, and your doctor doesn't take the time to ask you himself what the problems are, then that's a red flag that he's having to move too quickly to really do the "best" by you.

If you need to test this theory to prove that it's true, next time you're in a doctor's office where the nurse asks what's wrong, and you tell her the story like you usually would—notice how *little* she writes down. And then if the doctor isn't coming in and asking for all the details, make sure you say to him "there's more that I need to tell you."

Another problem with this approach is that if the nurse listens to you and then writes down things in *her* own words, then that can set the doctor up for an error in diagnosing your illness. Why? Because authorities on making correct diagnoses say that *why* you've come to the doctor that day (what in doctor-jargon is called "the chief complaint") should be *restricted to what the patient says*, and it's best when it's in the patient's *own words.** This is important because if the nurse writes down things in "her own words," *she* is doing the interpreting and diagnosing that the doctor should be doing, and that has the potential of unintentionally leading the doctor down the wrong diagnostic path. Don't think "oh, I bet that really happens rarely." It is a *common* cause of misdiagnosis. Don't let it happen to you.

(This type of misdiagnosis is caused by "error due to inheriting someone else's thinking,"* and this particular error causes the doctor to lean toward a particular diagnosis "as a result of a judgment *made by [another] caregiver* early in the patient care process."*)

If you're caught in a situation like this, and you have a medical condition that seems serious or is not getting better, just make certain that you repeat to the doctor the main reason you've come in, and then *all* of the things you said to the nurse, so he's certain to hear them.

It can also be a good idea in offices like this to say *as little as possible* to the nurse about your illness—just enough to give your main symptom and satisfy her. When the doctor comes in, say "I need to tell you more about what's going on," and then do so.

This is a good idea because it's hard to tell the same story twice and remember to put in all the details, and you're giving yourself the best shot at a correct diagnosis when the doctor is hearing all of the small details that may not, from the nurse's viewpoint, have been important enough to write down.

Remember that this advice is especially important if you have a recurring problem or symptoms that just don't seem to be going away. And remember to follow this advice if you have to be seen in an emergency room, where you almost always have to talk with the nurse first.

You could also bring a "Patient-Doctor Encounter Form" with you and give it to the doctor so that he has the history and symptoms of your illness right there in front of him, *in your own words*.

A "Patient-Doctor Encounter Form" can be downloaded from www.CautiousPatient.org.

*Campbell, Samuel G., Pat Croskerry, and William F. Bond. "*Profiles in Patient Safety*: A 'Perfect Storm' in the Emergency Department." *Academic Emergency Medicine* 14(8) (2007): 743-749, *italics added*. The particular diagnostic error described here is called "triage cueing."

Have more than one illness to discuss?

• If you go to a doctor's appointment with more than one problem that you want discussed or solved, it is very important that you *either* bring a list of what you want to discuss with him and give it to him at the very start of your appointment when he first comes in *or* tell him at the start of the interview that you have *x*-number of things to discuss, and here's what they are.

Have an extra copy of the list if you can, so that you can read down it with your doctor.

Having this written list, or telling the doctor at the outset that you have several concerns, is very important for several reasons.

One is that your doctor needs to schedule his time with you wisely, so he needs to know *at the outset* what your expectations are for that visit. There is almost nothing a doctor hates more than finishing up his visit with you, and then you saying "oh, and also ...."

And, if you bring up all of your concerns at the outset, then the doctor will have the opportunity to make an intelligent decision about how the time with you should be spent.

He may not be able to get to all of your concerns that day, and that's okay—you need to be aware that that is a possibility; but at least he knows what they are, and if any are life-threatening or health-threatening, he will be able to pick those off of the list and get to *them* that visit. Give him that opportunity.

You might even say, *at the beginning*, "I have *x*-number of concerns, and I know you might not be able to get to all of them today, but I want to tell you what they are." Then do so.

Then if there's something you especially need that day, tell him which one that is, and then he will also pick out any that might be health-threatening—again, give him all the problems at the outset so he has the data he needs to prioritize. Be prepared that he might ask you to come back another time for the other concerns.

Your doctor will be so appreciative that you are organized in this way, and are not one of the “and also” patients. And you will get better care when your doctor has all the data and can organize his time wisely.

Chronic illnesses aren't adequately managed by doctors more than 40% of the time

• You have been seeing your doctor regularly for some time now, and he is watching your diabetes, or blood pressure, or cholesterol, and you're taking the medicine he gives you, and you're doing whatever blood tests he asks. So everything's fine, right?

No.

It's hard to believe, but many chronic illnesses like high blood pressure, diabetes, heart disease and asthma are *not being treated adequately by doctors.*[3] Yes, the doctor is treating you, but over 40% of the time, the doctor is not treating you *adequately*, so that you can avoid early death or disability due to these problems.[3]

There are several reasons for this. Our healthcare system doesn't pay your doctor any differently if he treats you partially or if he treats you adequately for your illness. You don't know enough about how you should be treated, so you can't complain. Also, there are big problems with how the insurance companies and government insurers pay primary care practitioners (your family doctor, general practitioner, or general internist) for the time they spend with you, so often your doctor feels like he's doing the best he can with the time he can spend on you.

But that's not good enough. How are you going to avoid blindness, kidney disease, heart disease and amputations from poorly-controlled diabetes? Or a heart attack from years of having poorly-controlled blood pressure or cholesterol? Maybe you're one of the almost 55% who gets treated correctly. How are you to know?

You have to learn more about your illnesses. *You* need to find out what the recommended national guidelines are for your condition. You need to see what your lab results, blood pressure or medicines *should be*, and then compare them with *your* lab results, blood pressure, or medicines.

Sure, it's not what you'd like. You'd like the doctor to just take the time and thought to make sure that your chronic diseases are adequately treated.

But that's not happening for patients over 40% of the time. (More than 4 out of every 10 patients are not getting the treatment they should.)

If you find from the national guidelines that your numbers are not optimal, then take the national guidelines to your doctor and ask for more medication or other treatment that will bring your numbers into correct control of your condition. *But*

if you feel it would be really awkward to show up with national guidelines (that the doctor might not know about, and might make him really defensive), then just go in and ask for what you want. For example, if your blood pressure is 145/90 (but the guideline says it should be under 140/90), then just say "I'd like my blood pressure to be under 140/90. What should I take to get it there?"

Some doctors are going to have less of a problem with this approach because you're not challenging their authority or knowledge. If they ask "why," you can just say that you've read some things and that's what you'd like it to be.

The point is that you need to get the right care, and you need to think of some way to get it done without offending the doctor—which really doesn't get you anywhere.

Another thought is to play good cop—bad cop with your doc. Bring along your spouse, loved one, or whomever, and *he* can be the one with the national guideline who wants you to get your numbers in line, because *he* wants you to stay healthy and live longer.

You only have two choices: leave things like they are and suffer the consequences of complications and earlier death from your chronic disease—or go outside your comfort zone and use whatever measures seem most appropriate to get your doctor to help you get your disease adequately controlled.

If the advice in this section just seems way too uncomfortable for you to follow, then keep reading, and you'll find other information that will help with your health that's not as hard. Of course, taking all of this advice would be best, but you can only do what you feel comfortable with. And maybe a little down the road, you'll feel comfortable enough to try some of these harder bits of advice.

Following the national guidelines for your condition and making a flow sheet to make sure you're treated adequately is a lot of work, and, unfortunately, your doctor usually doesn't have the time. Since you are the one most interested in your health, you need to take it upon yourself to make sure that you get the adequate treatment you need.

There will be a day when most doctors appreciate your taking this initiative, and appreciate the help you're giving them. (It just probably won't be tomorrow.)

See more information on how to get the national guidelines and how to make sense of them at www.CautiousPatient.org.

"We calculated that comprehensive high-quality management of 10 common chronic diseases requires more time than primary care physicians have available *for all patient care* [more than 10 hours per day] … Our data show that there is not enough time for primary care physicians to deliver the services currently recommended for chronic disease management."*

*Ostbye, Truls, Kimberly S.H. Yarnall, Katrina M. Krause, Kathryn I. Pollak, Margaret Gradison, and J. Lloyd Michener. "Is There Time for Management of Patients with Chronic Diseases in Primary care? *Annals of Family Medicine* 3(3) (2005): 209-214, *italics added*.

Acute illnesses often aren't managed well either

• Many acute illnesses aren't managed well either,[3,*] and in certain situations, that can be life-threatening. But you can intercede in some ways to ensure better care.

For example, a study by Berger et al. showed serious quality problems in patients getting the care they should when they are hospitalized with a heart attack. The researchers studied eight "quality indicators" that patients should receive, if indicated for their particular type of heart attack and other illnesses or problems. They found that the patients received the indicated, recommended best care only 41% to 87% of the time.[†]

Some of the treatments were *so* basic, and yet 100% of the patients did not get the treatment. For example, in the patients that *should* have gotten aspirin during their hospital treatment for a heart attack, only 87% got that treatment.[†]

Now that may seem like a good percentage to some people, but if my loved one was in the 13% group who *didn't* receive this simple but life-saving therapy—I mean, how hard is it to order an aspirin a day when the American Heart Association has recommended that it be given during the hospitalization, and studies have shown that "the use of aspirin resulted in a 22% lower odds of 30-day mortality rate after adjustment was done for other variables."[†]

Twenty-two percent lower risk of dying in the first 30 days after your heart attack if you receive aspirin during your hospital stay, and yet 13% did not get that protection![†]

So, although you're not a doctor, here's what you can do in this situation to help your loved one.

If your loved one has a heart attack, the first day that he's in the hospital, go to the Cautious Patient website at www.CautiousPatient.org and search for "Quality Indicators," then look for "Heart Attack." Then take that list of treatments or medications to your loved one's doctor, and say, for example, "If John is a candidate for any of these treatments, then I want to make sure he gets them."

Take the list, and go down it with the doctor. For example, "Is John a candidate to take aspirin in the hospital?" If yes, then "Is he on it?" If no, then "Would you make sure he gets that?" Go on down the list.

You can ask that the doctor make your request part of the patient's chart.

Don't be obnoxious, but don't be shy either—you could save your loved one's life. Just let the doctor know that you want to make sure that *your* loved one gets 100% of the best care that he could.

(Although I gave you the example of 13% of heart attack patients didn't get aspirin when they should have, in 5 of the 8 quality indicators in the study, greater than 30% of patients did not receive the treatment or medication that they should have![†]) (Aspirin was just easiest to explain here.)

(In addition, although all 4300 patients in this study were eligible for at least one of the quality indicator treatments, 12% of the patients received *none* of the quality recommendations![†])

Yes, you're not a doctor, and it would just be so nice to be able to leave it up to the doctor. I mean, he's the one with all the training, and who are you to say what should happen?

But at these rates of non-compliance in ordering recommended medications or treatments that save the lives of patients with heart attacks, do you want to rely just on faith that your doctor is doing all that he can?

He may need a little help from you.

Additional quality indicators for other acute illnesses will be listed at www.CautiousPatient.org. Search for "Quality Indicators" at that website.

"The failure to use effective therapies for [heart attack] may lead to as many as *18,000 preventable deaths each year.*"[†]

*Bodenheimer, Thomas. "The American Health Care System: The Movement for Improved Quality in Health Care." *New England Journal of Medicine* 340(6) (1999): 488-492.

†Berger, Alan K., Daniel W. Edris, Jeffrey A. Breall, William J. Oetgen, Thomas A. Marciniak, and Gaetano F. Molinari. "Resource Use and Quality of Care for Medicare Patients with Acute Myocardial Infarction in Maryland and the District of Columbia: Analysis of Data from the Cooperative Cardiovascular Project." *American Heart Journal* 135(2) (1998): 349-356, *italics added*.

Whoa! Is it possible that doctors don't always follow the "best practice" guidelines that national organizations like the American Heart Association put out?

• It's not only possible, but usual.

Our medical system is so decentralized. Each doctor diagnoses diseases and treats patients based on what he was taught in medical training, and then catch-as-catch-can throughout his career as (and if) he reads journals or goes to medical conferences.

There's no centralized authority that says "Doctors! Look here! This is now the best set of treatments for a heart attack. Use it starting now!"

There's no "one" journal that says "Doctors! If you read this journal, you can stay completely caught up with the best practices!"

There are no bulletins from government offices that say "Alert! Here's a new and proven protocol to use to save the lives of more of your heart attack patients! Update how you do things—use these suggestions 100% of the time they're indicated!"

The time needs to come when doctors are helped to achieve more consistent and quality care. But for now, you'll have to help your doctor and your loved one the best you can.

Learn more about what how you can help at www.CautiousPatient.org.

It's up to *you* to make sure things get done correctly for you and yours.

"It is distressing to health care researchers that so much of the evidence they produce *remains unheeded in day-to-day practice*."*

"Each year clinical research produces new findings that may contribute to effective and efficient patient care. Although considerable resources are spent on undertaking this research, *relatively little attention has been paid to ensuring that its findings are actually implemented in routine clinical practice* ... The slow and haphazard process of translating research findings into clinical practice compromises the potential benefits of clinical research."†

*Hayward, Robert S.A. "Clinical Practice Guidelines on Trial." *Canadian Medical Association Journal* 156(12) (1997): 1725-1727, *italics added*.

†Grol, Richard, and Jeremy Grimshaw. "Evidence-Based Implementation of Evidence-Based Medicine." *Joint Commission Journal on Quality Improvement* 25(10) (1999): 503-513, *italics added*.

Your doctor doesn't have time for a lot of research, so you need to do it

• Realize that doctors have busy schedules and aren't always up on the latest, best, and nationally-recommended guidelines on everything medical.

"Today, no one clinician can retain all the information necessary for sound, evidence-based practice. No unaided human being can read, recall, and act effectively on the volume of clinically relevant scientific literature."*

After your doctor has diagnosed you with an illness, if something doesn't feel right, then get more information about that disease on the Internet, and decide for yourself if that diagnosis fits.[4, 5]

If you have a chronic illness, like diabetes, heart disease, asthma or high blood pressure, do research yourself on reputable Internet sites about your disease.[5] See what the recommended treatments and guidelines are for your disease, and take a copy of the information on your next doctor's visit (or use the other strategies mentioned in the Chronic Illness section).

You should be a valuable partner in your healthcare.

You can find information about reputable websites at www.CautiousPatient.org. (In addition, the Cautious Patient organization is an online support group for those who have had medical errors, and for those who are in situations where they're trying to get good care and avoid errors.)

And when you're doing your research and reminding your doctor about what you need in medical care to stay safe and healthy, be aware that your family physician or other primary care doctor is usually trying to do the right thing by you, but has not been able to figure out how that can be done, considering that the healthcare system's approach to family physicians is really dysfunctional—but that's an issue too big for this book.

You can just let the doctor know that you know he's trying, and you're just going to help when you can.

"*Patient-consumers are valuable reservoirs of largely untapped manpower.* Increasing dignity is being given to the patient's role, as well as greater appreciation for the complexity of patients' responsibilities. The person with a chronic disease, for example, functions at times as a nutritionist, lab technician, pharmacist, and nurse, capable of making some medical judgments."†

"Physicians have always had a professional obligation to base their decisions on the best available information ... The disappointing reality, however, is that *physicians still don't regularly search the medical literature themselves* ... Physicians don't, and never will, have that kind of time to look for the answers to most of their clinical questions themselves."‡

*Institute of Medicine. *Crossing the Quality Chasm: A New Health System for the 21st Century*. Washington, D.C.: National Academy Press, 2001, p. 25.

†Fischbach, Ruth L., Antonia Sionelo-Bayog, Annette Needle, and Thomas L. Delbanco. "The Patient and Practitioner As Co-Authors of the Medical Record." *Patient Counselling and Health Education* 1980 (First Quarter): 1-5, *italics added.*

‡Davidoff, Frank, and Valerie Florance. "The Informationist: A New Health Profession?" *Annals of Internal Medicine* 132(12) (2000): 996-998, *italics added.*

Worsening or changing symptoms after you've seen the doctor

• At the end of every office visit, when the doctor tells you what you have, and what he's going to do, he should *always* add "but if things change, or symptoms get worse, then come back in, or if the office isn't open, go to the emergency room."

Why? Because when you get a symptom or symptoms, then see the doctor, and he examines you and makes a diagnosis, the truth about medical care is that "that's what it looked like *then*." It's a "working diagnosis."

An illness can start out looking like one thing (maybe something basically harmless), and then end up being something else (maybe something that needs urgent attention). *Too much* respect for the doctor's opinion, on what is called the "working diagnosis," can be harmful, and even *deadly* to the patient.

For example, if a child starts with a stomach ache and vomiting, and sees the doctor, the doctor might diagnose a stomach virus, and give something for those symptoms until the virus runs its course. But if the child goes home and starts running a fever and the abdominal pain gets *worse*—then what looked like a stomach virus that morning, could look like appendicitis that afternoon.

And appendicitis that is not adequately treated with surgery can be deadly.

So, *never* think that when you've gotten the diagnosis from the doctor, then that's exactly what it is, regardless of what happens next. If nothing changes and you've got a good doctor, then you're probably fine.

But if anything changes or gets worse, or you don't get better on the time-table that the doctor gave, then you *must be* re-examined—for your safety.

Read more about misdiagnosed or undiagnosed conditions when you get to Endnote 4.

"Once a diagnosis has been established, it is often used [by doctors] to explain all newly occurring symptoms *without necessarily considering* that another underlying disease might be present."*

The Kirch and Schafii study quoted just above noted that one of the reasons for misdiagnoses is that a doctor doesn't rethink his position. And that can be a medical error that is sometimes fatal. Since that is a common error that doctors make, *you* need to keep an open mind, and insist on re-evaluation if things change, get worse, or symptoms don't go away.

*Kirch, Wilhelm, and Christine Schafii. "Misdiagnosis at a University Hospital in 4 Medical Eras: Report on 400 Cases." *Medicine* 75(1) (1996): 29-40, *italics added.*

Beware of the "it's-all-in-your-head" diagnosis

• In so many of the cases of misdiagnosed or undiagnosed illness, the patient is worked-up by the doctor, and when nothing is found that he can diagnose, he tells the patient "it's all in your head" (or words to that effect).

Most of the time, it's *not* all in your head. So when you hear the "it's all in your head" diagnosis from a doctor, it's usually best to interpret that as an "I can't figure out what's wrong with you" diagnosis.

It's not always the fault of the doctor that he can't diagnose what's wrong. Several things could be going on that are beyond his control.

Most commonly, what happens is that many serious diseases present insidiously—a little at a time. And the first symptoms of the disease may not trigger even the best doctor to be able to figure out what it is.

So it's vitally important that your doctor establish an ongoing dialogue with you in cases where he can't figure out what's going on. He should say "I can't really tell what this is right now. We should watch it—many times these things go away. But if they don't go away, or if you get more symptoms, then we need to re-evaluate you."

And then that's what should happen.

Many symptoms, especially if they're somewhat low-key in terms of severity, just go away, and we *don't know* what caused them. We didn't invent the human body, and we haven't spent a lot of research money trying to name and diagnose illnesses that go away on their own.

Other times, those are the first symptoms of disease, but the disease hasn't progressed far enough along for the doctor to be able to diagnose it. And sometimes your symptoms aren't the typical ones for a certain disease, so it takes longer to figure it out.

In any case, it's important for both you *and* your doctor to keep an open mind, and re-assess if things change, become more severe, or just don't go away.[4, 5]

In rarer situations, even if your doctor is a good one, what's happening could be something rare that he hasn't seen or even heard of.

In this case, if your symptoms aren't too severe or urgent, it's usually okay to wait to see if they persist. And if they do, and your doctor still can't diagnose what's wrong, then ask him what kind of specialist might be able to look at your symptoms more closely, and then go forward with a specialist.

All of this is not to say that stress (maybe that's what those doctors are referring to when they say it's all in your head) can't cause a lot of symptoms. Stress can and does cause a significant number of physical symptoms and can make you more susceptible to many illnesses.

But most people can tell when the diagnosis of "stress" fits and when it doesn't. Keep alert and follow your intuition.

"A wealth of research shows that patients thought to have a psychological disorder ["it's all in your head"] get short shrift from internists and surgeons and gynecologists. As a result, their physical maladies are often never diagnosed or the diagnosis is delayed."*

"Misdiagnosis sometimes results from a failure to listen to what the patients say about their symptoms, *or dismissing their concerns too hastily* ["it's all in your head"]."†

*Groopman, Jerome. *How Doctors Think.* New York, New York: Houghton Mifflin Company, 2007, p. 39.

†Vincent, C.A., and A. Coulter. "Patient Safety: What about the Patient?" *Quality and Safety in Health Care* 11 (2002): 76-80, *italics added.*

Misdiagnosed

• If your doctor has made a wrong diagnosis, then obviously your treatment is going to be incorrect, and you're not going to get better. And plenty of misdiagnoses continue to be made.

> "There is now abundant evidence that *delayed or missed diagnoses are widespread* and that in more than 50% of such cases there are serious adverse outcomes."*

There is a wealth of new information about thinking and decision-making mistakes that doctors can fall into when they're deciding on a diagnosis.[4]

Dr. Jerome Groopman describes what often happens:

> "On average, a physician will interrupt a patient describing her symptoms within eighteen seconds. In that short time, many doctors decide on the likely diagnosis and best treatment. Often, decisions made this way are correct, *but at crucial moments* they can also be wrong—with catastrophic consequences."[†]

It's obvious that these snap judgments aren't always the best way to properly diagnose patients, but doctors haven't really been taught how to keep their minds open to other possibilities.

Borrell-Carrio and Epstein discuss "low-level" thinking that doctors often use to make diagnoses, and give some examples of these incorrect, low-level thinking patterns.[‡] Do any of these sound like your doctor?

1. "I've got it! As soon as the patient told me, I knew what he had."[‡]

2. "If the patient is satisfied with the diagnosis of another physician, why should I bother to find out more data?"[‡]

3. "When in doubt, choose the simplest or most convenient hypothesis."[‡]

4. "[Patient] complains a lot? He doesn't have anything!"[‡]

Higher-level thinking involving the same 4 situations above would be:

1. "I should look beyond early hypotheses [assumptions]."[‡]

2. "I should always form my own criteria."[‡]

3. "When in doubt, assume the worst hypothesis."[‡]

4. "I must take a fresh look."[‡]

Borrell-Carrio and Epstein believe that doctors should be taught to use high-level decision rules in thinking, and to be taught to examine their thinking, to see if they are falling into lower-level decision-making traps.[‡]

The most common cause of misdiagnosis is what is called "premature closure."[§] In this scenario, the doctor just closes his mind to any new alternatives once he's decided on a diagnosis. As you'll see in several later sections in the book, this can be very dangerous for the patient.

But what can you do when doctors use these low-level thinking patterns and don't re-think their original diagnoses?

You need to understand that this can happen, so that you don't take every word that comes from doctors as if it were gold. And since doctors often can't spot their mistakes, then you need to give some direction when you feel things aren't right. You need to be able to say "that doesn't sound right," or "I'm not getting better and I want us to re-think this," or "something just isn't right—what other tests do we need to see if it's something different?"

Sometimes it's even necessary to seek out a different doctor and present your case as "new"—so many times if a doctor hears the previous diagnosis, he just closes his mind and you don't get a fresh look.

And, as noted in a previous section, you may need to do your own research.

Am I suggesting that you question every diagnosis from your doctor? No. But *do* question the diagnosis when you feel something isn't right, when things aren't getting better, or when things seem to be going downhill fast.

*Croskerry, Pat G. Letters: "Prescribing Powers for Pharmacists." *Canadian Medical Journal* 176(1) (2007): 67, *italics added.*

†Groopman, Jerome. *How Doctors Think*. New York, New York: Houghton Mifflin Company, 2007, p. 39, *italics added.*

‡Borrell-Carrio, Francesc, and Ronald M. Epstein. "Preventing Errors in Clinical Practice: A Call for Self-Awareness." *Annals of Family Medicine* 2(4) (2004): 310-316.

§Graber, Mark L., Nancy Franklin, and Ruthanna Gordon. "Diagnostic Error in Internal Medicine." *Archives of Internal Medicine* 165 (2005): 1493-1499.

Medications: prescribing errors

- Tragic errors can be made in prescribing medications.[6,*]

"Studies have shown that 15% to 21% of prescriptions contain at least one prescribing error."[†]

Sometimes the doctor doesn't remember your drug allergies; sometimes he's not considering the other drugs you are on; sometimes the doctor's handwriting is poor; many times the doctor isn't recalling the right dosage and frequency for the medication he's prescribing.

In one medical study, mistakes in dosing (the strength of the medication) caused 54% of the errors, and mistakes in frequency (how often to take the medicine) caused 18% of the errors made by doctors in prescribing medicines.*

Sometimes, having the doctor "call in the prescription" produces errors more often because some drugs "sound like" others, and some dosages are misunderstood over the phone.

Errors made in prescribing medications can be hard for the patient to avoid. But there are definite steps that you can take to protect yourself.

The first thing to do is to remind the doctor of any drug allergy you have as he is handing you your prescription. Say, for example, "You remember that I'm allergic to penicillin, right?" Don't just trust that he'll always remember to look.

Next, make sure that you can clearly read the name and dosage of the medication on the prescription. If you can't, then ask the doctor, and print the drug name, dosage, and how to take it more clearly right on the prescription itself, even if you have to do it yourself. Pharmacists hate to have to guess about what medication the doctor is prescribing, but pharmacists also seem to get a lot of grief from some doctors when they call to get clarification.[‡] So it's better if you just make sure yourself before you leave the doctor's office. *Don't skip this step!* If you're feeling uncomfortable, blame it on your pharmacist if you have to: "How do you spell this? My pharmacist always asks me when I hand in my prescriptions." Just get it done.

Next, when you get home with your new prescription, plug the name of the drug into a website like www.drugs.com. Once you pull up the medication, click on one of the "Consumer Information" links. The "Med Facts" or "Concise" link will tell you what the medication is for—here you can check to be sure that the medication matches your condition the doctor is using it for. Then look under "Detailed" or "Advanced" to make sure that the dosage and frequency of the medicine as your doctor prescribed it is within the recommended guidelines. *Don't skip this step either.* And if you find a discrepancy, make sure you talk with your doctor before you take the medication.

Your neighborhood pharmacist could be very helpful. If you have the same pharmacy filling all of your prescriptions, and if they know your allergies, they can catch many of the prescribing errors there.

Pharmacists are also usually really friendly and willing to answer questions. And if they're busy right then, and you want to ask some questions, just ask them when they might have more time, and they'll tell you when they are usually slow and can answer more of your questions.

In addition, elderly patients (those 65 years and older) are at increased risk for medication problems,[§] and it has been shown that elderly patients are often prescribed drugs that they really shouldn't be taking.[6] Check at www.CautiousPatient.org for these medications under "Medications Contraindicated in the Elderly." Then check with the doctor if a loved one 65 years or older is on one of these medications, and see if it can be safely discontinued. Better safe than sorry.

> "In our study [of adverse drug events in outpatient care], most of the preventable events were due to prescribing errors (an inappropriate choice of drugs, drug interaction, or drug allergy)."*
>
> "Lines of communication between the pharmacist and the physician are fragmented as a result of the pharmacist's hesitancy to contact physicians and because of physician inaccessibility."[‡]

*Gandhi, Tejal K., Saul N. Weingart, and Joshua Borus et al. "Adverse Drug Events in Ambulatory Care." *New England Journal of Medicine* 348(16) (2003): 1556-1564.

†Gandhi, Tejal K., Saul N. Weingart, and Andrew C. Seger et al. "Outpatient Prescribing Errors and the Impact of Computerized Prescribing." *Journal of General Internal Medicine* 20 (2005): 837-841.

‡Brown, C. Andrew, Jessica H. Bailey, Joshua Lee, Paula K. Garrett, and William J. Rudman. "The Pharmacist-Physician Relationship in the Detection of Ambulatory Medication Errors." *American Journal of the Medical Sciences* 331(1) (2006): 22-24.

§Gurwitz, Jerry H., Terry S. Field, and Leslie R. Harrold et al. "Incidence and Preventability of Adverse Drug Events among Older Persons in the Ambulatory Setting." *Journal of the American Medical Association* 289 (2003): 1107-1116.

Medications: side effects and medication interactions

• Realize that most doctors can't possibly know all the side effects of all the drugs they prescribe, *or* how all those drugs might interact with each other. And studies report that most doctors still don't use an electronic drug-checker to check for reactions between your drugs (drug-drug interactions).*

"Physicians do not routinely screen for potential drug interactions, even when medication history information is readily available."*

You can go to a website made for non-medical people like www.drugs.com to see if some new symptom could be caused by your medication. (Once at the website, plug in your drug, then search, then scroll down to "Consumer Information" to look at what you should know about the drug, including side effects that even your doctor might not be aware of.)

Let your doctor know if you find something important.

You can also plug *all* of your drugs into the "Drug Interaction Checker" at www.drugs.com, and it will alert you if there are any interactions between the medicines. Let your doctor know right away if you find any.

Yes, you'd think that 21st century medical care would have had that done before you were given the prescription—but it doesn't. Thank goodness you can do it yourself!

*Institute of Medicine. *To Err Is Human: Building a Safer Health System.* Linda T. Kohn, Janet M. Corrigan, and Molla S. Donaldson, eds. Washington, D.C.: National Academy Press, 2000, p.39.

Medications: lab tests are often needed for safety *before starting* and *while continuing* certain medications

• Drugs are toxic as well as helpful. Although the proper dosage of medication improves health and saves lives, the improper use can cause tragic outcomes.

When some drugs are used, it is recommended that the doctor measure your blood count, kidney function, liver function, or electrolytes *before* starting the medicine. This is because that particular drug is known to affect that body system, and the drug manufacturers and FDA think that doctors should know if that body system is working properly before you start a drug that might affect it detrimentally.

Unfortunately, many doctors forget to do this. A recent study by Raebel et al. found that 39% of the time, drugs are prescribed without the recommended initial lab testing.*

Also, there are recommendations on how your body systems should be monitored for possible damage when you take certain medications on a long-term basis. Unfortunately, this recommended monitoring doesn't always happen either, and this omission could seriously harm your health. Hurley et al. report that "lapses in laboratory monitoring of patients taking selected chronic medications *were common*,"† and, of all adverse drug reactions, "monitoring errors were the cause of 60.8% of preventable events."†

With estimates of over 700,000 patients per year being treated in U.S. emergency rooms for adverse drug reactions, and over 100,000 people hospitalized per year for drug reactions,‡ it may be time for you to get involved so that you can save yourself or a loved one from this harmful and sometimes deadly problem.

Checking to see if you need certain lab tests before or while you're on a certain medicine is a little difficult, but you should still be able to manage it. Again, go to a website like www.drugs.com and type in your drug, but this time click on "For Professionals." Then go down to the "Warnings" or "Precautions" section. If there are certain tests that should be done before or during your use of that medicine, they should be listed there. The only problem is that this information is in "doctor-speak," so it may be more difficult for you to figure out. Here are a few suggestions.

Your friendly pharmacist may come in handy. You might ask him if there are any warnings or recommendations of lab tests that should be done before or during use of that medication.

Or, if you find something at www.drugs.com that mentions tests to be done before or during the use of that medicine, call your doctor and mention that you found these lab tests that can be helpful, and ask him to order them for you.

Also, you can find a list of some common drugs that need monitoring at www.CautiousPatient.org, along with tests that should be done.

Now, you may be thinking "this is all too much. I don't have time for all this." Okay. But just remember that you *can* double-check these things, and do it when you have a feeling that things just aren't right.

*Raebel, Marsha A., Ella E. Lyons, and Susan E. Andrade et al. "Laboratory Monitoring of Drugs at Initiation of Therapy in Ambulatory Care." *Journal of General Internal Medicine* 20 (2005): 1120-1126, *italics added.*

†Hurley, Judith S., Melissa Roberts, and Leif I. Solberg et al. "Laboratory Safety Monitoring of Chronic Medications in Ambulatory Care Settings." *Journal of General Internal Medicine* 20 (2005): 331-333, *italics added.*

‡Budnitz, Daniel S., Daniel A. Pollack, Kelly N. Weidenbach, Aaron B. Mendelsohn, Thomas J. Schroeder, and Joseph L. Annest. "National Surveillance of Emergency Department Visits for Outpatient Adverse Drug Events." *Journal of the American Medical Association* 296(15) (2006): 1858-1866.

Medications: just plain mix-ups

• Another thing that often goes wrong is that a person's medication gets really mixed-up.

A family doctor gives some medication for one or more conditions. Then the patient might have to go to the emergency room, and gets another prescription there. Then he sees a specialist—maybe an eye doctor, or a foot doctor, or a cardiologist—and other medicines are prescribed. Then maybe the patient goes to a drugstore clinic on the weekend for a minor illness and gets more medicine. And maybe the patient is taking a few supplements from the health food store that the doctor isn't aware of.

Sometimes, even when a patient is only seeing *one* doctor, the doctor might add a new drug, but also means to tell you to stop taking another, but either you or the doctor forgets. Maybe the doctor decided to switch you from one medication to a similar one that he thought would suit you better, or maybe he decided to change the dosage of the prescription. Either way, there you are with a new prescription, and it hasn't been made perfectly clear to you that you shouldn't still be taking all those that you still have at home!

What can happen in these cases is that patients often end up taking several different drugs that are essentially in the same drug class, but the combination of the two is not needed, and can be harmful. Or the patient is taking drugs that, combined with the others that they're taking, could be harmful and potentially fatal.

To make sure this problem doesn't happen to you or yours, be sure to go to Appendices A and B and use a personal health record to keep all your medicines up-to-date, neat and printed, so that when you see the doctor, he can scan the list easily and make sure they're the right ones to be on. Those handwritten lists just aren't as easy to scan, so make sure you use the medication page of the personal health record.

And when *any* doctor gives you a new prescription, then hand him your printed-out current medication list, and ask him if there are any that he wants you to now discontinue. This advice is so important—don't forget to do this.

(In addition, this will give the doctor one last look at your current medications, and he'll be more likely to catch his own error if he is prescribing something new that he sees might interact with something on your list.)

Test results: no news is *not* good news

• You've done your job—you've seen the doctor and had your pap smear done, or your lab work done, or your x-ray done, and now you're waiting for the call to tell you what the results are.

Here's the problem: many doctors don't have their practices organized in a way that makes it certain that they get all the test results back, and that they follow up on all abnormal results.

So you're waiting a while, maybe even make a call or two to the office, but when you don't hear back, you assume everything's okay, and go on about your life.

But this assumption can be dangerous.

> "There is growing evidence that the failure to follow-up on abnormal test results is a common medical error that can compromise patient safety."*

And after you've been discharged from the hospital or the emergency room, studies have shown that abnormal test results that are reported after you left *may never reach you.*

> "Approximately 6% of patients hospitalized in a major academic medical center had ... [important, abnormal] test results return after their discharge *without the knowledge of the responsible physician.*"*

If you're going to follow-up on tests in order to be sure that you get the abnormal results (should there be any), then you're going to need to know what tests are being done. So when you're checking out at the front desk, ask what lab tests were done, and write them down, so that *you* can make sure you get results.

And when you get the results, do yourself and everyone else a favor and get a copy of them *right then.* Then later, when some doctor's wondering about what was done, you'll have the answer.

If you're in the office when the lab results come back, then ask for a copy of them right then. If you're getting the results over the phone, then ask them to fax you a copy "for your records."

It's not a lot to ask, and is vital to your good health.

One tip: most of the time doctors don't want patients to have copies of their lab reports because they don't want to have to explain each and every test (some blood metabolic panels include over twenty different "tests"), and/or explain every minor abnormality. Be realistic—most doctors don't have time to explain all these things to you. Just let them know that you just want a copy to keep a complete record. If there's some hesitation, you might even say "I just want a copy for my records. If I need to talk about them further, I'll make an appointment."

Please understand how vital it can be to your good health to have these lab results available. Doctors feel so frustrated when you go to the emergency room, or a walk-in clinic, or your regular doctor, and you say "they (wherever) did some blood tests and said everything was fine." We don't ever want to hear that. To give you the best care, we want to know *what* tests, and *what* the results were.

And just don't make any assumptions about your test results. Make sure you make a note to follow-up on them, and never assume that "no news is good news."

*Sung, Sharon, Valerie Forman-Hoffman, Mark C. Wilson, and Peter Cram. "Direct Reporting of Laboratory Test Results to Patients by Mail to Enhance Patient Safety." *Journal of General Internal Medicine* 21 (2006): 1075-1078, *italics added.*

The problem with after-hours phone calls to your out-of-the-office doctor

• Although it is very comforting to be able to call your doctor when the office is closed, know that you probably don't have his full attention. He may be sleeping, drinking, or driving, and his full attention is not on you like it is when you are in the office.

So be very cautious when relying on medical advice you get over the telephone. It's a double-edged sword. When you get it, you feel better. But is it really reliable?

The doctor hasn't seen and examined you. He's relying on you to convey medical information. Since you have no medical training, he's most likely offering an opinion based on incomplete information.

In addition, when you call doctors when they're not in the office, they're likely to be less focused—more distracted. To be safe, you must use your intuition in seeking medical care.

Definitely, if you have sudden severe and continuous pain, or you see a condition in a loved one that has worsened and now worries you, go to the emergency room and get a valid examination and opinion.

If you're calling with a quick question, then sometimes that's fine. But if it is a new illness or a question about something getting worse, or anything that takes more than a minute to explain, you really need to take your loved one to the emergency room and not rely on the doctor to reassure you that it can wait until morning.

Many fatal mistakes have been made by doctors reassuring scared patients that they can wait until morning, no problem—but the doctor didn't get all of the story because he couldn't see the patient, and he was not sharp and focused on asking all of the right questions that might have protected the patient.

Several recent studies have confirmed this point.

In a 2007 study, Katz et al. described 32 cases of telephone-related medical malpractice claims.

"The most common allegation was failed diagnosis (68%); [the] most common injury was death (44%)."*

"Faulty triage" was an error in 84% of the cases "usually because of incomplete history taking over the phone."* ("Triage" is deciding the seriousness of the medical situation—whether someone needs immediate attention, or whether it can wait.) The doctors did not "guess right" about whether the illnesses were serious or not *in 84% of those malpractice claims.*

Of the 32 patients described above, *fourteen died.*

"Regarding faulty triage decisions, a dynamic seems to emerge when medical complaints are presented over the phone compared to seeing patients in the office. *Evaluation is more difficult on the phone* because of time pressure, as well as not being able to see the patient during the dialogue. As a consequence, history taking is often rushed and incomplete, letting the patient, rather than the clinician [doctor], do the triage."*

See Endnote 7 for a case in point and results of another study.

If you think your loved one is in medical trouble, then call 911 if urgent, or take them to the emergency room where a doctor can see them right away.

Don't be a statistic—doctors can't diagnose through the phone, or when they are sleepy or focused on other things.

*Katz, Harvey P., Dawn Kaltsounis, Liz Halloran, and Maureen Mondor. "Patient Safety and Telephone Medicine: Some Lessons from Closed Claim Case Review." *Journal of General Internal Medicine* 23(5) (2007): 517-522, *italics added.*

Your after-hours call to a doctor to see if you should go to the emergency room—your doctor might have conflicting loyalties

• Be aware that when you call a doctor when he's not in the office, and you give him your symptoms and ask his opinion—do you need to go to the emergency room, can he call something out, or can it wait until office hours tomorrow—his advice *may* be influenced by how his managed care contracts pay him.

Many managed care contracts monetarily penalize doctors if their patients show up in emergency rooms, and expend the managed care money in emergency room expenses. Unfortunately, sometimes your symptoms *need* emergency care.

What to do? It's a hard call, but in order to stay safe in our dysfunctional system where the doctor is also trying to play by managed care rules, you need to know all of these factors that your doctor *may* be using to make his decision, so that you can protect yourself and your family.

So, you must use your own good judgment here, and seek emergency care when you think you need it, regardless of what the doctor has said.

Don't be a statistic. Your intelligence and intuition were made for you to use and to protect you.

"The capitation-plus-bonus-payment mechanism [paying doctors more when they hold down payments on services like emergency room visits] attempts to control medical care costs by appealing to the economic concerns of physicians ... [This type of payment] *may encourage the physician to wait rather than to act.*"*

*Bodenheimer, Thomas S., and Kevin Grumbach. "Capitation or Decapitation: Keeping Your Head in Changing Times." *Journal of the American Medical Association* 276(13) (1996): 1025-1031, *italics added.*

Phone calls to the doctor when he is in the office

• When you call a doctor's office to get a question answered by your doctor, make sure that the answer comes from your doctor, and is not just the opinion of the nurse. Much of the time, if the nurse just answers the question on the spot, then the answer is suspect.

Many doctors allow their nurses or office personnel to answer questions like this because they just don't feel they have the time to do it themselves.

To make sure that you're getting the right information, you should ask "would you just check that with the doctor when you have time and give me a call back?" Maybe add "my case is a little different."

Better safe than sorry. Most good doctors want the questions to go through them first. Just little variations in symptoms or questions can cue a doctor that something is amiss—something that a nurse might not catch.

And realize that the same issues and dangers from "after-hours phone calls to your out-of-office doctor" also pertain here. (You may not be giving the complete medical information needed for him to give the best advice, and he is probably focused primarily on the patients *in* his office.)

I've seen tragedies where the patient has called and talked with the doctor in the office, but because the doctor wasn't actually examining the patient, he didn't understand the seriousness of the situation, and tragedy occurred.[7, 8]

Just be aware of the risk, and you'll be better off.

Breast lumps

• Be aware that breast lumps are treated in a different fashion from doctor to doctor, and the inconsistency that exists is very conducive to a patient becoming a victim of a late diagnosis of breast cancer, when there is a much higher rate of dying.

Notably, failure to diagnose breast cancer has been the leading or second most common reason for malpractice suits in many recent years.

Many people believe that if they have a breast lump and the mammogram is normal/negative, then they're fine.

Nothing could be farther from the truth. Mammograms are only 70 to 85% accurate in diagnosing cancer in women with a breast lump.

If you have a breast lump and a normal mammogram or ultrasound, be aware that a third tool is available to help make the right diagnosis, and that tool is a needle biopsy.

When you add the needle biopsy to the mammogram and the clinical breast exam (palpation done by a doctor), experts call this the "triple assessment protocol," and many believe that this is necessary for you to have the *best* chance at an early diagnosis of breast cancer.

So, to protect yourself: if you have a breast lump that has persisted for more than one or two months, *even if you have a negative mammogram,* consider insisting that your doctor use a needle biopsy to make a more accurate diagnosis.

You can go to the Internet and search with the words "breast triple assessment" for more information.

There have been too many mothers, daughters, sisters and friends who have died from breast cancer that could have been diagnosed and treated if it had been caught earlier. Don't let that happen to you.

"We found that *a substantial proportion* of women with a breast problem managed by generalists *did not receive care consistent with a clini-*

cal guideline, particularly younger women with a clinical breast complaint and a normal or benign-appearing mammogram."*

"Problems with breast cancer can include underuse of mammography for early cancer detection, *lack of adherence to standards for diagnosis (such as biopsies and pathology studies)*, inadequate patient counseling regarding treatment options, and underuse of radiation therapy and adjuvant chemotherapy following surgery."†

"Mammography screening is far from perfect ... Mammography does not depict all cancers."‡

"Every radiologist who has any long-term experience has failed to perceive something of importance that is visible in retrospect ... All radiologists, no matter how skilled or dedicated, cannot avoid periodically missing a clinically important lesion."‡

*Haas, Jennifer S., E. Francis Cook, Ann Louise Puopolo, Helen H. Burstin, and Troyen A. Brennan. "Differences in the Quality of Care for Women with an Abnormal Mammogram or Breast Complaint." *Journal of General Internal Medicine* 15 (2000): 321-328, *italics added.*

†Institute of Medicine. *Crossing the Quality Chasm: A New Health System for the 21st Century*. Washington, D.C.: National Academy Press, 2001, p.24, *italics added.*

‡Kopans, Daniel B. Editorial: "Mammography Screening Is Saving Thousands of Lives, But Will It Survive Medical Malpractice?" *Radiology* 230(1) (2004): 20-24.

You may not be getting the tests or the specialty referral you need for your medical condition—divided loyalties

• If you take a look at the national treatment guidelines for your chronic medical condition, like diabetes or heart disease, you may find that you're not getting all of the lab tests that you need to get.

And some of you may be going to your doctor repeatedly for a condition, you're not getting any better, and yet your doctor isn't referring you to a specialist.

Be aware that some insurance companies pay doctors, or even decide whether a doctor can be in their "network," by whether or not the doctor holds down the amount of money he spends on tests and specialty referrals. In some financial arrangements, doctors try to hold down those testing and referral numbers so that they can get the full payment offered by the managed care organization (MCO). (Some are called health maintenance organizations or HMOs.) The MCO withholds a certain portion of the doctor's payment, and then the doctor's "bonus" at the end of the year depends upon how well he holds down costs on testing and referrals.

Although it's unfair to patients for their doctors to have these divided loyalties, these are the facts in medicine today.

Your doctor is likely to have patients in several different insurance plans. For example, in a contract with one company, for that group of patients he might get paid a set fee each time they come in for an office visit. In a contract with another company, for that group of patients he gets paid a certain amount per month for each of those patients, no matter how many office visits they need. And in a contract with still another company, he also gets paid a certain amount for each of those patients per month, but lab fees, x-rays, and referral fees (to specialists) have to be paid by *him*. That insurance plan pays that way on purpose—to encourage the doctor to order only what's required.

I guess it's only human nature that *some* doctors let it color their decisions when it comes to you.

What doesn't feel fair is that you, the patient, don't know what the doctor's financial arrangement is *for you.* It seems only fair that doctors should disclose to you what their financial arrangements are with *your* insurance company, so that you could make your decisions wisely by knowing all the facts. Or maybe your insurance company should disclose that information to you.

Maybe we could get disclosure of the financial arrangements when we check in at the reception desk—so that we know when our doctors have these divided loyalties. Or maybe it could be posted on the wall at the office.

I guess it's reasonable that insurance companies want to pay doctors like this—they are trying to hold down the cost of medical care. But shouldn't you get to know if your doctor has that kind of financial relationship in *your* situation? It seems only fair.

In the meantime, make sure that you know what tests you need for your chronic condition and make sure that you're getting them. And if you're seeing your doctor and not getting better, *insist* that he refer you to a specialist.

"Many managed-care organizations include financial incentives for primary care physicians ... Incentives that depend on limiting referrals or on greater productivity apply selective pressure to physicians in ways *that are believed to compromise care.*"[*]

"A spectrum of methods exists for calculating physician bonus payments. Each physician's referral costs may be tracked individually, with the end-of-year bonus depending on each physician's own cost to the IPA in specialty and ancillary referrals."[†]

"Primary care gatekeeping, in which *the goal of the primary care physician is to reduce patient referrals to specialists and thereby reduce costs*, is not an adequate system in which to practice medicine ... The practice of primary care is troubled ... Most managed care organizations use primary care physicians as gatekeepers, controlling access to specialty care."[‡]

"Many believe physicians are still placed in situations that create potential conflicts of interest ... Patients currently have little knowledge of these implicit rationing methods that can affect access and the types of care they receive."[§]

And as a matter of public policy:

"With their high levels of administrative expenditures and executive compensation, health maintenance organizations have skimmed billions of dollars from the healthcare economy."**

*Grumbach, Kevin, Dennis Osmond, Karen Vranizan, Deborah Jaffe, and Andrew B. Bindman. "Primary Care Physicians' Experience of Financial Incentives in Managed-Care Systems." *New England Journal of Medicine* 339 (1998): 1516-1521, *italics added.*

†Bodenheimer, Thomas S., and Kevin Grumbach. "Capitation or Decapitation: Keeping Your Head in Changing Times." *Journal of the American Medical Association* 276(13) (1996): 1025-1031.

‡Bodenheimer, Thomas S., Bernard Lo, and Lawrence Casalino. "Primary Care Physicians Should Be Coordinators, Not Gatekeepers." *Journal of the American Medical Association* 281(21) (1999): 2045-2049, *italics added.*

§Cleary, Paul D., and Susan Edgman-Levitan. "Health Care Quality: Incorporating Consumer Perspectives." *Journal of the American Medical Association* 278(19) (1997): 1608-1612.

**Bodenheimer, Thomas. Education and Debate: "Disease Management in the American Market." *British Medical Journal* 320 (2000): 563-566.

Referrals to specialists: your doctor's advice may be tainted by your insurance plan

• Doctors in today's marketplace don't always have the option of just giving you their best advice. Even though they should be primarily looking out for *your* interests, many times today they're caught in a bind between what they *would like* to recommend (and what they would do *for their own family members*), and what your medical plan *allows them* to recommend.

This conflict-of-interest imposed by today's healthcare system is terrible for patients and for the consciences of doctors as well.

Nevertheless, it's a reality, so you need to know it.

One of the places this can be most troublesome is when you're seeing your primary care physician (family doctor or general internist) and he needs to refer you to a specialist to have something looked at or taken care of that's outside his area of expertise.

Sometimes when he pulls out and looks at the list of specialists who are in your plan, he experiences an inward groan. He knows that he wouldn't pick any of those doctors to treat any of his loved ones, and he's not happy about sending you to one of them either.

Doctors, after a period of time in practice, *know* which other doctors they'd use for themselves, their family members, and recommend to their friends, because those specialists have shown themselves to be honest, kind, trustworthy, and proficient.

Others, for example, may be kind but not proficient; proficient but somewhat dishonest; honest, proficient and kind, but seem to have a substance abuse problem or aren't always reliable; honest and kind, but don't keep up with the latest recommendations and developments very well.

You, the patient, are the one in the real bind, and you never even know it's happening.

So, when your doctor refers you to a specialist, take that referral name, and then ask him, confidentially, if there's another name that he could recommend—someone whom he'd send his own mother or child to, even if that doctor is not in your healthcare plan. Just tell him that you might also want to take a look at that doctor.

And please, especially when you're being referred to a specialist who may be doing a procedure or operation on you, really check to make sure you're seeing someone who is well-experienced and well-thought-of in that specialty and that procedure. Board-certification, which is so highly-touted by so many, is *not* a substitute for a recommendation from a real, living person, preferably a doctor you trust, as to who's a good, safe specialist to go to.

If you're in a plan where you can see other doctors but you have to pay a little more when they're not "in network," then if you're referred to that doctor from a reputable source—*that's money well spent.* Doctors aren't interchangeable—if you get a referral from a reputable source, then you're best off going to that specialist for your care.

And, to avoid some problems in the first place, if you have any choice at all, *don't* allow yourself to be in a healthcare program that *absolutely* limits whom you can and can't see.

Your healthcare *plan* can affect your health

• Healthcare plans come in about three general types: (1) those where you can see any doctor you want (often called fee-for-service); (2) those where you can see any doctor you want, but the insurance company will pay less if the doctor you pick is "out-of-network" (not in their plan) (often called a PPO); and (3) those where they won't pay *at all* for your care unless you use in-network doctors (often called an HMO).

If you're able to choose your healthcare program, pick the first or second option whenever possible.

And only choose the third option—only being able to choose in-network doctors—if you absolutely have no other way to get health-care.

Why? Because your best option at getting good medical care is to be able to see a specialist or other doctor who has been recommended to you by a trusted friend or other doctor. And if one of those recommended doctors is not on the HMO list, then you may be just picking a doctor in total darkness.

Your HMO only checks to see if the doctor has the right "credentials" and "specialty certification." Unfortunately, those alone don't guarantee that you get a good doctor.

> "The various accreditation and licensure programs for health care organizations and providers [physicians] have been promoted as 'Good Housekeeping Seals of Approval,' yet they *fail* to provide adequate assurance of a safe environment. Reducing medical errors and improving patient safety are *not* an explicit focus of these processes."*

So if you have a choice of healthcare plans, don't choose a plan where your choice of doctors is absolutely limited. And if it's the only way you can get healthcare, then just keep your wits about you and remember that the HMO approval or specialty accreditation only goes so far.

*Institute of Medicine. *To Err Is Human: Building a Safer Health System.* Linda T. Kohn, Janet M. Corrigan, and Molla S. Donaldson, eds. Washington, D.C.: National Academy Press, 2000, p.43, *italics added.*

Do the best you can to stay with the primary physician of your choice

• Any insurance plan that doesn't allow you to see the primary physician of your choice is a terrible waste of resources. Doctors are *not* interchangeable. You and your doctor forge a relationship over time, and the skill of the doctor whom you've chosen and *knows you* just can't be easily replicated.

Medical care is not like fixing flat tires in an assembly-line fashion. So much time is spent over months or years that informs the doctor on who you are, and he *uses* that information as he treats you. That time and history just can never be recovered when you are forced to change doctors because of a job change or a health plan change. And that personal relationship can be critical to your diagnosis and treatment.

Try not to ever sign up for an insurance plan that doesn't allow you to stay with your trusted physician.

I guess insurance companies just look at doctors like auto mechanics—interchangeable. (And many people would argue that auto mechanics aren't interchangeable either!) The doctor that you've seen regularly, or even several times, knows more about you than what your medical records reveal. He is often more like a friend or confidante. Think of yourself when you meet someone new like a minister or a teacher. At first both of you are somewhat wary—who is this person? Then over time, you both decide if you "fit"—if you like and trust each other enough to have a satisfactory relationship. Doctors and patients are like that.

When your family doctor, whom you trust and who knows you, is seen as interchangeable with any other family doctor, that's a big problem for you and our entire healthcare system.

How in the world did we get to a place where healthcare organizations don't know this!

(In addition to the above, think about the amount of time and resources it takes for any doctor to see a "new" patient, and get up to speed on all of the unique medical features that make up that particular patient—what a waste of time and resources!)

"Those who have studied trust say that it develops through a series of encounters wherein one party demonstrates 'trustworthiness' to the other ... The Medical Outcomes Study revealed a disturbing trend toward declining physical health in these vulnerable populations [the elderly and the poor] who were enrolled in a health maintenance organization [HMO] rather than in a private practice [where they could choose their own physicians] ... The profession as a whole should adopt a standard that encompasses the concept that physicians should maintain and cultivate long-term, trusting relationships with their patients."*

*Branch, William T., Jr. Commentary: "Is the Therapeutic Nature of the Patient-Physician Relationship Being Undermined?" *Archives of Internal Medicine* 160 (2000): 2257-2260.

Asthma treatment

• Asthma is an old condition that has very good therapies now. The asthmatic patient can, many times, completely control his symptoms with a step-wise use of the new medications.

I hate to see parents who feel so panicked and vulnerable because they often have to rush their child in because of an asthma attack, when the child's asthma could be well-controlled with a little time and good medical management.

If you or your child are an asthma patient who makes frequent trips to the doctor's office or emergency room for out-of-control symptoms, then go to www.CautiousPatient.org to find the most highly-recommended asthma treatment protocol. Print out that protocol and take it on your next doctor's visit and ask that the protocol be followed until you are under control.

The deaths from asthma, and they still happen, can often be prevented by the use of peak-flow meters, which are very inexpensive (about $20). *Every* asthma patient should have one on hand—it's a lifesaver, and the only way a serious asthmatic can know exactly how much trouble he's in, and get emergency care if needed, before it's too late.

Asthma patients are particularly sensitive to errors caused by medication mix-ups. Re-read the "Medication: just plain mix-ups" section, and make sure you follow that information very carefully if you are an asthma patient.

"To improve asthma disease management, the National Asthma Education Panel (NAEP) Expert Panel ... published *Guidelines for the Diagnosis and Management of Asthma*. Although the NAEP guidelines were published 7 years ago [when this study was done], compliance with the guidelines was low. It was especially poor for use of preventive medication and routine peak-flow measurement."*

*Legorreta, Antonio P., Jennifer Christian-Herman, Richard D. O'Connor, Malik M. Hasan, Reaburn Evans, and Kwan-Moon Leung. "Compliance with National Asthma Management Guidelines and Specialty Care." *Archives of Internal Medicine* 158 (1998): 457-464.

Procedures and operations: studies show a lot of inappropriate use

• Realize that if a doctor is pressuring you into a procedure, *scaring you* into a procedure, or discouraging you from getting a second opinion, that is your cue to get out of there.

A reputable doctor will always respect your intelligent decision to get another opinion, or to look at the literature or do some Internet searching before you decide on a procedure.

If the doctor proposes doing a procedure on you there in his office, be aware that some studies have shown that there is a substantially increased risk of complications and death in procedures done in a doctor's office versus those done in outpatient surgery centers.*

Studies have also shown that many surgeries or procedures are undertaken when *it is inappropriate to do so.*[9] And all of these surgeries or procedures have a level of risk involved.

> "A number of studies have demonstrated overuse of health care services; for example, from 8 to 86% of operations—depending on the type—have been found to be *unnecessary and have caused substantial avoidable death and disability*."†

Leape et al. studied coronary artery bypass surgery in New York State, and found that some patients received the surgery *who were not appropriate candidates.*[9] Considering that we're talking about heart surgery, it's certainly not something that someone should have done unless it was absolutely indicated.

A study by Chassin et al. across eight states found coronary angiography, carotid endarterectomy, and upper GI endoscopy used *inappropriately* in 17%, 32% and 17% of patients, respectively.[9]

(Coronary angiography is when the doctor threads a catheter to your heart to shoot dye into the arteries that feed the heart, so he can see those arteries better. Carotid endarterectomy is an operation done on the arteries in your neck when they have narrowed considerably. GI endoscopy is where the doctor puts a tube down your esophagus to look into your stomach.)

As you can imagine, anytime you're dealing with catheters that go to your heart, or surgery that involves blood supply to your brain, you are at risk of complications. Obviously, no one should undergo these procedures without good reason.

GI endoscopy has risks as well.

And Bernstein et al.'s studies found that 16% of hysterectomies and 4% of coronary angiographies were performed for inappropriate reasons.[9]

Some families have seen their loved one harmed or die from a procedure or operation that they later found *did not need to be done.*

So anytime that you're advised by a doctor to have a procedure or operation, keep your eyes open, and check, check, and re-check before you agree to do it.

*Vila, Hector, Jr., Roy Soto, Alan B. Cantor, and David Mackey. "Comparative Outcomes Analysis of Procedures Performed in Physician Offices and Ambulatory Surgery Centers." *Archives of Surgery* 138 (2003): 991-995.

†Bodenheimer, Thomas. "The American Health Care System: The Movement for Improved Quality in Health Care." *New England Journal of Medicine* 340(6) (1999): 488-492, *italics added.*

Procedures and operations: think before scheduling

• Understand that when you are going to a consult in the office of a doctor who derives a great proportion of his income from procedures or operations, *for some* of those doctors there just seems to be a natural inclination for them to go right to "well, we need to set you up for …"

It's almost as if it's a given, that if you show up in that specialist's office, that you must want the surgical/procedural option. But usually, they are really supposed to be *evaluating* your condition to see if you *need* a procedure for further diagnosis and/or treatment.

You really need to do your research here before you go right to the scheduling of the procedure. And if you can get a referral from a really trusted source to a specialist that doesn't always go directly to procedures, then that might be a better place to start.

Too many times, I've heard from a friend who has taken himself in to see some specialist, and then phones me after to say "I saw the [*name of specialist*] today and he said the MRI (or hemorrhoids or arthroscopy or other test) was one of the worst he's ever seen!" And then my friend tells me that he's already gotten the doctor to schedule the operation (or procedure), so that he can get it fixed right away.

There seems to be some sort of tight connection between "it's the worst he's ever seen" to "I'm going to get this taken care of right away." And something about the "it's the worst" phrase seems to cause them to lose objectivity about getting a second opinion or doing some checking on their own.

And I know that there are medical ways to solve many of those problems, and I know that when my friend gets done with the surgery—well, things could be fine, but things could be worse. There are possible complications with any procedure or operation. And then when you're in a post-surgical state, where your body is irreversibly changed, and if you're not better, then you can't turn back time from that.

So I try to give my friends a little heads-up warning.

And for you—just be careful. Look at non-surgical alternatives and do your homework before you schedule a procedure or operation.

Some doctors are "bad apples"

• Realize that doctors are not always what they seem. Just like in any other walk of life, there are some bad apples in the barrel, and they can be just as friendly and professional-looking as the good apples.

If you find your doctor doing something "just a bit dishonest," it's probably just the tip of the iceberg. Go elsewhere.

Just follow a general policy of keeping your eyes wide open, following your instincts, and not trusting in doctors as if they were gods or infallible.

Some "bad apple" doctors run kind of a "racket" where they use non-standard therapies to bring the patient back to the office over and over again (for repeat charges, of course), or have a "treatment" that patients might not be able to get somewhere else. You might ask your doctor "is this a standard treatment for [*your condition*]?"

If the answer is no, then don't see this doctor again. If the answer is yes, *then verify it* by looking it up on the Internet.

And some "bad apple" doctors run a racket where they get all their specialist friends to evaluate the patient—of course, this racket usually only works where insurance is paying the bill, and I've only seen this racket in hospital situations. But this type of racket is really paid for by all of us, and many times patients go through procedures that don't need to be done—such a waste of resources as well as the discomfort the patient might have to undergo with unnecessary evaluations.

The "injection" racket

• Here's the scenario: Patient gets sick. Patient goes to doctor. Doctor listens, examines, and says "the nurse will be in to give you a shot. I'll leave a prescription at the front desk." Patient gets shot. Patient leaves, thankful that he's seen this fine doctor who found that he was so sick that he needed a shot. He's reassured that he'll be well soon—I mean, he got a shot!

But here's the problem—the patient doesn't really *need* a shot, and by ordering one, the doctor makes more money.

And there's no way for the patient to realize that the shot wasn't actually necessary.

So, ironically, the patient walks out of the doctor's office, after taking an *unnecessary* hit in his gluteus *and* wallet, actually thinking, "Wow, it's a good thing I came in. I guess I was so sick I needed a shot!"

Here is the real truth about shots (injections): you almost never *need* an injection to get well. For most illnesses, an injection doesn't do anything that a prescription medicine won't do. In almost all cases, after you get the shot, you *still* need a prescription anyway. And as soon as you take that first dose of your prescription—you're on the same road to recovery.

And even for those illnesses like strep throat or poison ivy, where an injection will actually completely treat the illness, there are medication equivalents that could be used instead of the injection. Okay, if the doctor orders an injection here, the patient *would* be cured—but wouldn't it be fairer to offer that decision to the patient? ("I could give you a shot for this, or a prescription that you'd need to take for a week—which would you prefer?")

But I don't want to get distracted by those really rare occasions where the injection is actually curative, because *most of the time*, the shots are just completely unnecessary—just ordered to give the doctor something tangible to do, and, by the way, increases his profit.

No medical school teaches doctors to use shots like this, and there are no medical books that advise using shots in this fashion.

I think this shot racket is especially offensive when the recipient of the shot is a child. Those kids are so frightened—if the shots were *necessary*, it would be okay to give them, but when they aren't needed—I mean, where are the hearts in these docs?

And I've seen it done in children. I've seen pediatricians who give vaccines to children much more frequently than any national organization recommends. I've seen doctors give children monthly shots of immune globulin "to help them not get sick." (There is no reputable organization/book/school/whatever that recommends doing this.)

Sometimes $100 shots. And higher. And for working people without insurance. And for our ailing healthcare system. How can these docs really justify this?

I've seen medical clinics where the doctors had to order a certain number of tests/injections/whatever *to keep their jobs*. (It's a kind of "you want fries with that" or "do you want the extended warranty" approach, but without the consumer getting to make the decision.)

Yes, there are *some* instances where it's appropriate to give an injection. When the patient is nauseous or vomiting, an injection might be indicated.

Of course, most doctors don't run this "racket"—just be aware that this is a problem you may run into. If your doctor *does* like to give shots—well, it all depends on how easy it is to find a doctor where you live who doesn't. What you may need to do with a doctor who prescribes a shot is say, "I don't want a shot. I want to take a prescription."

Then, if the shot isn't really needed, you might see the doctor back off some.

And for those of you who like getting those shots—well, I guess if you're happy ... But just be aware that when you get your prescription filled, you're going to get just as much good from your first dose; and by getting that shot, you *are* increasing the cost of healthcare.

And you who don't get unnecessary shots from your doctor—be glad that your doctor is taking the high road instead of prescribing you a profitable placebo.

Our medical school professors would be so disappointed in us if they knew that things like this, that we were never taught, are *learned* out here in the real world, where there's no one here to look over our shoulders and shut us down when we're going down the wrong path.

Note: Unnecessary *antibiotic* injections seem to be the most common. Unnecessary *steroids* run a close second.

Stuck with a ccrtain doctor or clinic?

• Some people are in a certain healthcare plan that they're stuck in—it's the only one their employer offers; it's the only one that the government offers; it's the only one in the area; or it's the only one they can afford.

If you are in a tough situation where you *must* use a particular doctor or clinic, and you don't think you are getting the care you need or deserve, then you might need to take a particularly assertive action to get what you need.

Government HIPAA (pronounced "hip'-uh") regulations say that you have a right to see your medical records—so ask your doctor's office for a copy of them and look through them. The very least you should be able to see is if your doctor has written down what you came in for, the symptoms you told him, what his assessment was (the reason for the symptoms or the diagnosis), and what his plan was to treat your illness.

As hard as it is to imagine, some doctors don't write down the symptoms and concerns you tell them.* It's almost like if they don't write your symptoms down in the chart, then they don't have to spend time to do anything about them.

(I've actually seen this happen too frequently. Think of it: if the patient is harmed by the medical care [or lack of it], and wants to bring a malpractice claim, then the doctor just points to the records: "See, I didn't know he had such-and-such-symptoms. He didn't tell me.")

If your doctor is not putting your symptoms into the chart, or if you're not getting the answers that you need or your symptoms still aren't diagnosed, then at your next visit, bring a "Patient-Doctor Encounter Form" that you have filled in with what you want your doctor to know about your condition that day, and what questions you have for him. See www.CautiousPatient.org for this form.

Ask your doctor to make that form you've filled out part of your medical record.

(Federal HIPAA law *requires* doctors to allow patients to amend their charts, so that would be a reasonable request if you're in this situation. See the Cautious Patient website at www.CautiousPatient.org to get a copy of the HIPAA requirement that you can print out and take to your doctor if you need to, to show him that it allows you to amend your chart when it is incorrect or incomplete.)

Once that becomes part of your record, then the doctor is on notice that he needs to do something about it. You should get better care then.

*Pakhomov, Serguei V., Steven J. Jacobsen, Christopher G. Chute, and Veronique L. Roger. "Agreement between Patient-Reported Symptoms and Their Documentation in the Medical Record." *American Journal of Managed Care* 14(8) (2008): 530-539. This study found disagreement "between patient self-report [of symptoms] and documentation of symptoms in the medical record."

Preventing illness

• Do your family a favor and get the preventive medicine tests that you need.

For children, this usually means immunizations and checks for proper growth and development.

For women, it usually means pap smears and mammograms at certain ages and recommended intervals.

For all adults, it means having your blood pressure and cholesterol checked from time to time.

For adults over 50, there are a few other tests that you should start getting.

And for all, the tests that you need often depend upon your own medical history and your family health history.

But again, you can't just leave it up to your doctor to tell you what you need. An interesting but alarming 2003 study concluded that each family physician would need an additional 7.4 hours per working day *just providing preventive medicine* if he were to fully satisfy the recommended preventive guidelines for his patients!* So you can imagine that you're not getting the complete picture if you just leave it to your doctor to remember to give you all the recommendations.

Find out what the national guidelines are for preventive medicine at www.CautiousPatient.org.

"Poor compliance with recommended schedules of clinical preventive services is a well-documented problem in primary care. The good intentions and usual resources of providers are often insufficient to carry out satisfactory clinical prevention … One major reason for this may be that … [the physicians] *fail to involve the person with the most to gain from the clinical prevention effort: the patient.*"†

"The increasing role of managed care, with its emphasis on increased productivity [number of patients seen per session], appears at odds with primary care physicians' increasing responsibility for prevention."‡

"Preventive services consensus goals are not being met, even for patients who report that their clinic visit was for a checkup or physical examination ... Perhaps the most concerning pattern to emerge from these data is that even for patients who reported visiting the clinic for a checkup or physical examination, the grand mean at which indicated preventive services were prescribed was *only 46%*."§

*Yarnall, Kimberly S.H., Kathryn I. Pollak, Truls Ostbye, Katrina M. Krause, and J. Lloyd Michener. "Primary Care: Is There Enough Time for Prevention?" *American Journal of Public Health* 93(4) (2003): 635-641.

†Dickey, Larry L., and Diana Petitti. "A Patient-Held Minirecord to Promote Adult Preventive Care." *Journal of Family Practice* 34(4) (1992): 457-463, *italics added*.

‡Stafford, Randall S., Demet Saglam, and Nancyanne Causino et al. "Trends In Adult Visits to Primary Care Physicians in the United States." *Archives of Family Medicine* 8 (1999): 26-32.

§Kottke, Thomas E., Leif I. Solberg, Milo L. Brekke, Antonio Cabrera, and Miriam A. Marquez. "Delivery Rates for Preventive Services at 44 Midwestern Clinics." *Mayo Clinic Proceedings* 72(6) (1997): 515-523, *italics added*.

Your doctor as an indcpendent individual—an "autonomous" individual—and how that affects you

• This concept is important for you to understand so that you can take the steps you need to get around this "fluke" in medical care. (Some would say "flaw.")

Autonomy, the ability to do whatever you want with little or no oversight, has always been an important part of the medical profession. A doctor is taught to use his training in the basic and clinical sciences to formulate diagnoses and treatments that he, individually, thinks are the best. This was probably a good idea when there were no nationally-recommended guidelines and few proven strategies to reduce complications and deaths from certain illnesses. And it's probably also been a needed part of medicine because many people have combinations of diseases and allergies and the doctor needs to be able to *think* what the best thing is for that particular patient, given everything he knows about medicine and the patient.

Certainly, when I was in medical school, we were directed to *not* use any kind of checklist approach to patient care. We were to look at each patient individually and then, remembering anatomy, physiology, biochemistry, microbiology, pathology, pharmacology, etc., we were to diagnose that patient and formulate a treatment plan. This probably made sense in those simpler days, before we had the massive amount of research that we now have, that shows us very scientifically what should be done as treatment guidelines for many illnesses, and preventive guidelines to prevent disease.

Now it's different, and we do have these guidelines. But some doctors just don't like it—they're used to doing things the way they want. They're used to being "autonomous"—and they like it like that. They grumble, and call it "cookbook" medicine, and don't want to be held to the standards that "other people" have laid down as best medical practices.

But there are other problems that this "autonomous" attitude causes. One is a problem with being part of a "team" and treating nurses and other hospital personnel with respect, and we'll get to that later.

But the problem I want to deal with now is that, because of this autonomous "I'll-do-what-I-please" attitude, it has been shown that some doctors will resist efforts to make them "play by the rules." And if the rules are for *your* best interest, then that's a problem for you.

One researcher found that when doctors were ordered by hospital administrators to follow policies relating to patient safety, "there was a common lack of support for the hospital's new safety systems."*

The researcher continued, "As with previous studies in this area, my findings highlight the potential for doctors to resist, subvert and capture managerial prerogatives in order to maintain professional authority."*

And a few more studies/articles along these lines:

> "Doctors may not necessarily regard guidelines as legitimate or identify with the rules written for them by members of other social groups … Advocates of standardization … view doctors as rule breakers."†

> "Physicians stoutly resist real or perceived efforts to curtail their independence, including the behavioral changes required to improve quality."‡

Another study found a problem with doctors failing to enter needed information into an electronic record at the hospital to prevent drug allergy reactions.

> "Clinicians often failed to enter allergy information into the computer regularly when patients had had allergic reactions during hospitalization, and the medications *were ordered again for the patients.*"§

In that study, they found that doctors actually entered that necessary allergy information *only 16% of the time.*§

So now that you know what you may be dealing with, you may be better able to figure out how to get what you need from doctors.

But equally important is for you to understand what you *will not get.* Since each doctor does things "his way," and some doctors just sort of refuse to follow the rules set by others, then *you* need to take the initiative to get the care you need and to keep some of your most important medical information accessible and up-to-date.

And that brings us to the next topic: Problem Lists.

*Waring, Justin. "Adaptive Regulation or Governmentality: Patient Safety and the Changing Regulation of Medicine." *Sociology of Health & Illness* 29(2) (2007): 163-179.

†McDonald, R., J. Waring, S. Harrison, K. Walshe, and R. Boaden. "Rules and Guidelines in Clinical Practice: A Qualitative Study in Operating Theatres of Doctors' and Nurses' Views." *Quality and Safety in Health Care* 14 (2005): 290-294.

‡Blumenthal, David, and Charles M. Kilo. "A Report Card on Continuous Quality Improvement." *The Milbank Quarterly* 76(4) (1998): 625-648.

§Bates, David W., Lucian L. Leape, and David J. Cullen et al. "Effect of Computerized Physician Order Entry and a Team Intervention on Prevention of Serious Medication Errors." *Journal of the American Medical Association* 280(15) (1998): 1311-1316, *italics added*.

You need a "problem list"

• The "Problem List" is a very important part of the medical chart that lists all of the following about a patient: drug allergies, diseases and conditions, hospitalizations, surgeries, important family medical history, important habit history (smoking, drinking, exercise), and important social history. Doctors are taught in medical school to keep an up-to-date problem list for every patient, and then, by looking at it, can easily become re-acquainted with the medical features of that patient that are important. When problem lists for each patient are kept complete, with an absolute attention to detail, they are incredibly valuable.

However, doctors don't get paid any better if they have a complete and organized problem list on each patient or if they just try to do their best, with the time that they feel they have to spend on each patient. At the frantic pace in today's healthcare, you can usually bet that your problem list is not as complete and up-to-date as *you* could make it.

The authors of one study stated "problem lists may contribute substantially to patient safety and quality of care" but "physician documentation of the problem list is often lower than desired.* They also noted that at one healthcare organization, "46% of the charts had an *empty* problem list."*

So, an accurate and up-to-date summary of your medical history is very valuable, but here's your problem—your doctor doesn't have the time to do it properly; or you're seeing more than one doctor, so you don't have *one complete* problem list; and/or your doctor or other provider just doesn't feel the need to make one.

> "The problem list is an important piece of the medical record … To enable its potential benefits, the problem list has to be *as accurate, complete and timely as possible*. Unfortunately, problem lists [at this healthcare facility] are *usually incomplete and inaccurate, and are often totally unused*."[†]

And in that healthcare facility, they were using electronic health records, so don't think for a minute that that will be the answer to all your medical record problems. It's just as easy for an electronic record to be incomplete and inaccurate as it is for a paper version.

Considering all of the above, do you really want to leave this vitally important summary of your health to someone else, or *anyone* else, when you can do it for yourself so much better?

You need to make and keep an up-to-date problem list.

Do you really want to take the chance that someone forgot to put your penicillin allergy into the problem list? How about your hysterectomy? If that isn't in the record where your doctor can find it, he could be giving you the wrong information about estrogen treatment. If your family history of breast cancer isn't where the doctor can easily find it, then you might not get the advice you need on when to start and how often to get mammograms. If your father's early heart attack isn't where doctors can readily see it, then your doctor's calculation of your cardiac risk will be incorrect, and you may not get the advice and drugs you need.

SO, even if we were at a place where all doctors had electronic records, I would trust the personal health history that the patient, *who cares the most that everything is right*, has prepared, over anything I see in a chart that someone else has prepared, whether it is in paper or electronic form.

And I've also seen medical charts prepared by doctors that had *wrong* information in them! A hospital record that says the patient had a history of high blood pressure—nope. And have you seen the scratch paper (and sometimes their palms) that many doctors write on when they're in a hurry? Please—not good for accurate transcription.

And when you're in the hospital and the doctor is there quizzing you about your health history, illnesses, surgeries, allergies, and symptoms—when he's not writing it down into the chart right then, but is getting the information so that he can go outside and dictate it or otherwise put your information into your record, do you really want to trust that it all gets into the record correctly?

Just say no. And then get yourself a personal health record that makes a problem list from what you've entered as your drug allergies, diseases and conditions, hospitalizations, surgeries, important habit history, and important social history. See Appendices A and B about making yourself a personal health record.

And take it to every doctor's visit, along with your medication list.

"Many EHRs (electronic health records) adopted by physicians to-date are missing basic features. Surprisingly, even simple functionalities such as *problem lists* or *procedure lists* were only available in approximately 8 of 10 EHR systems used by respondents ... Overall, many physicians are only partially adopting EHR technologies, suggesting that published adoption rates may be exaggerating the true rate of diffusion."[†]

*Galanter, William L., Daniel B. Hier, Chiang Jao, and David Sarne. "Computerized Physician Order Entry of Medications and Clinical Decision Support Can Improve Problem List Documentation Compliance." *International Journal of Medical Informatics* 2008, epub ahead of print, *italics added.*

†Meystre, Stephane M., and Peter J. Haug. "Randomized Controlled Trial of an Automated Problem List with Improved Sensitivity." *International Journal of Medical Informatics* 77 (2008): 602-612, *italics added.*

‡Menachemi, Nir, Eric W. Ford, Leslie M. Beitsch, and Robert G. Brooks. "Incomplete EHR Adoption: Late Uptake of Patient Safety and Cost Control Functions." *American Journal of Medical Quality* 22(5) (2007): 319-326, *italics added.*

The electronic medical record

• Even if your doctor has an electronic medical record (instead of the paper records that most doctors keep now), I want *you* to examine it periodically so that you know that the information in there is correct. Make sure that your allergies, medications, diseases, procedures and operations, and pertinent family history of disease are in there.

Keep in mind what you've learned about autonomous doctors. Keep in mind that doctors and other medical personnel are human and can make errors. Keep in mind that *you* are the person most interested in the health of yourself and your loved ones.

Remember that no one (not even doctors) can perform flawlessly. Remember that a too-tired, too-rushed, too-absentminded, or too-stressed doctor can easily make a mistake in your records that can set you up to be a victim of a medical error, a misdiagnosis, or just not achieving your best health outcome.

Remember that when data is in an electronic form that moves from doctor to doctor, if there's an error in the data that *any* doctor puts in, then *every* doctor who sees you will operate on that wrong information. Just as in financial records like credit reports, an electronic record can be much more efficient, but also much more of a pain when wrong information gets in there.

You are entitled to see and have a copy of your medical record; *but*, some doctors make it financially expensive to get a copy. If that is the case where you are, then ask that you be allowed to examine the record at the office. State medical boards have rules that doctors must follow to allow patients to see their records, even if they can't afford, or don't want to pay, for a copy.

At the very least, look at your problem list in the electronic record. Make sure that everything is complete and correct.

And if the electronic record doesn't have a problem list, then just keep bringing the one you have from your personal health record, along with your medication list, to every appointment with every doctor.

Electronic medical records can be an efficient resource, but *only* if patients, who care the most, make sure that the records are complete and correct.

One more thing: if our government decides to take matters into its own hands and gives us all electronic health records with links to our own personal health records, then that would be efficient and could be less work for you. The record would be somewhat transparent, so that you could see most of the data that doctors would be using to make decisions about your health.

If that happens and you don't have to be as much involved in your record and still get quality care, that's fine and good.

Just don't wait until that happens. These things take years to plan, years to implement, and years to fine-tune. Make sure you're involved in making sure your records are true and complete so you can start getting better healthcare *now* by making your own personal health record (see Appendices A and B), and checking your doctor's electronic record, if he has one, as described above.

But I don't want to have to participate this much in my medical care—I just want the doctor to do it

• We're talking about almost 100,000 hospitalized Americans dying each year as a result of medical errors, many more hundreds of thousands being harmed, plus all those who suffer harm or don't get good care as an outpatient.

Be sure and read Endnotes 1, 3, and 4.

And then if you still feel like leaving everything up to the doctor, then at least you know what your risks are.

Several surveys/studies have shown that most Americans don't really *want* to be involved in their healthcare—they'd rather let the doctor do the work and make the decisions.* As a result, well-meaning national organizations that work to improve the quality of healthcare just sort of throw up their hands—what are you going to do if people don't *want* to participate or help in their healthcare?

But it always occurs to me—what if the people answering those surveys *knew* what their odds of getting poor care or harmful care were? Sure, it'd be great if we didn't have to do anything ourselves; sure, we'd like to leave it all to the doctor. But who among you would do that for yourself or your loved one after knowing these statistics on undertreated, overtreated, mismanaged, and harmful care? I'd like to see the survey on *that*.

"Instead of treating patients as passive recipients of medical care, *it is much more appropriate to view them as partners* or co-producers *with an active role in their care* which needs to be recognized and enhanced."†

*Arora, Neeraj K., and Colleen A. McHorney. "Patient Preferences for Medical Decision Making: Who Really Wants to Participate?" *Medical Care* 38(3) (2000): 335-341.

†Vincent, C.A., and A. Coulter. "Patient Safety: What about the Patient? *Quality and Safety in Health Care* 11 (2002): 76-80, *italics added.*

Why haven't I heard of these things before?

• Many national agencies (the Institute for Healthcare Improvement, the Agency for Healthcare Research and Quality, the Joint Commission, and the National Patient Safety Foundation) know of the 100,000 lives lost every year in U.S. hospitals due to medical errors, and have been working for the last ten years or so to decrease harmful medical outcomes and improve the quality of medical care. They have worked mostly behind-the-scenes (out-of-sight of the American people) to solve quality problems by raising awareness and improving conditions in hospitals. They've undoubtedly saved many lives with their recommendations and the changes they've put into place in hospitals.

But there's a real disconnect between these agencies and the American public. Thus, *you* don't know there's this big problem, so you can't take steps to prevent these things from happening to you and yours.

There are probably several reasons why these governmental and other health quality agencies haven't alerted you in the same way that they would have if it was a deadly epidemic caused by something *other than* poor medical care.

Regardless of the reasons, the facts are that the American public has not yet felt the urgency of the situation. Maybe you've read some statistics, or heard some stories, or had a less than successful experience yourself with the healthcare system. But it has not been really impressed upon you that this is an epidemic, and we all have to participate to stop it.

Your awareness is vital to improving the situation.

To quote the Institute of Medicine:

> "*Public awareness* of shortcomings in quality is critical to securing public support for the steps that must be taken to address these concerns."*

"*The most important barrier* to improving patient safety *is lack of awareness* of the extent to which errors occur daily in all health care settings and organizations."†

"The 21st-century health care system envisioned by the committee—providing care that is evidence-based, patient-centered, and systems-oriented—also implies *new roles and responsibilities for patients and their families, who must become more aware, more participative, and more demanding* in a care system that should be meeting their needs."*

It's possible that those national organizations just don't quite know what to tell you, and don't want to create a widespread panic.

But I believe that what you don't know is really dangerous for you—and I think there are a lot of steps you can take to ensure better outcomes for yourself and your loved ones.

*Institute of Medicine. *Crossing the Quality Chasm: A New Health System for the 21st Century*. Washington, D.C.: National Academy Press, 2001, pp.7, 20, *italics added.*

†Institute of Medicine. *To Err Is Human: Building a Safer Health System.* Linda T. Kohn, Janet M. Corrigan, and Molla S. Donaldson, eds. Washington, D.C.: National Academy Press, 2000, p.157, *italics added.*

Your ability to stop medical errors *before* they can affect you

• If you want to avoid being a victim of a medical error, you have to participate.

Luckily, it looks like your participation is very helpful. In a study by Parnes et al., it was found that many potentially harmful events can be stopped *before they cause harm*—"stopping the error cascade"—by attentiveness, vigilance, and perseverance by the members of the healthcare team, including nurses, doctors, pharmacists, *and* patients and their families.*

> "Some people appear to have these characteristics [attentiveness, vigilance, perseverance] such that, in the presence of an error, there is a persistent sense that something is not right and it must be pursued until a satisfactory level of assurance is reached ... These characteristics may also be taught by cultivating a culture of safety: one that inculcates [stresses] attentiveness, safe questioning, and resolutions among clinicians, staff *and patients*."*
>
> "Importantly, we found that *patients* can also be effective ameliorators [persons capable of stopping medical errors before they affect patients]."*

But I know how hard it is for you to speak up, especially around doctors, when they have all the training, and you don't.

Leonard et al. describe how "hierarchy, or power distance, frequently inhibits people from speaking up," but "teaching people how to speak up and creating the dynamic where they will express their concerns *is a key factor in safety*."†

You can really make a difference in the safety of your care, if you care enough, and you speak up. Here's more advice from Leonard et al. on the best ways to speak up.

> "People need to state the problem politely and persistently until they get an answer; the common practice of speaking indirectly (the 'hint and

hope' model) is fraught with risk. Focusing on the problem and avoiding the issue of who's 'right' and who's 'wrong' is quite important and a major success factor."†

So follow their advice: speak politely and respectfully about what you need, and be clear about it. And don't get into power struggles about who's right or who's wrong—just focus on getting what you need in the simplest and least stressful fashion.

*Parnes, Bennett, Douglas Fernald, and Javan Quintela et al. "Stopping the Error Cascade: A Report on Ameliorators from the ASIPS Collaborative." *Quality and Safety in Health Care* 16 (2007): 12-16, *italics added.*

†Leonard, M., S. Graham, and D. Bonacum. "The Human Factor: The Critical Importance of Effective Teamwork and Communication in Providing Safe Care." *Quality and Safety in Health Care* 13 (Suppl. 1) (2004): i85-i90, *italics added.* The authors are speaking here of teaching nurses to speak up, but this advice applies as soundly to patients.

When you have some questions for your doctor ...

• Always go to each appointment ready to participate in a dialogue with your doctor. You'll get the best healthcare when you are a *participant* in the visit—*you* are the expert on you, and the doctor must have the information that only you can give him.

Be sure to ask any questions that you want to, need to, or feel would help you. Embody the attitude you want to see in your physician: kind and respectful. Oh, and also professional—*you* are the professional on you.

But if you leave the appointment feeling that your questions weren't heard or answered, think about this: your doctor, even if he's a saint, can have the following difficulties with answering questions:

- He may be a good doctor, but may be unable to communicate well "on the patient's level."
- He may be a good doctor, but just gets irritated when patients question him. (Some would argue whether or not this is a "good doctor," but we'll give him the benefit of the doubt here.)
- He may be a good doctor, but this just isn't a good day for him personally (family, finances, sleep loss, etc.).
- He may be a good doctor, but just doesn't feel he has the time to answer many questions from patients because of time and production pressures. (This is happening more and more with the bureaucratic hassles doctors have to attend to.)
- He may be a good person, but as a doctor, he just hasn't found the time to keep up with the best practices recommended in medical care.

And if your doctor is not giving you all the information you need, or not answering all of your questions, then use the other resources we've mentioned to find out more about your illness and treatment.

But make sure that you understand that one of the first strategies to use to get good care is to show up for your appointment ready to engage your doctor and participate in your care. It's not a safe option anymore to just sit back and be "a good patient." Effective healthcare requires the input and participation of both doctor *and* patient.

"There are at least two bodies of knowledge that are relevant to the exchanges between doctor and patients—the doctor's and the patient's. Both are experts in their own fields ... Caring for a patient requires both parties to recognize and respect the other's area of expertise."*

*Kennedy, Ian. "Patients Are Experts in Their Own Field: The Interests of Patients and Healthcare Professionals Are Intertwined." *British Medical Journal* 326 (2003): 1276-1277.

Odds and ends: advice and vaccine records

• Beware of relying on other medical people for serious medical advice.

Some medical tragedies have occurred because patients have asked *and relied on* nurses, paramedics, or other "medical" friends or acquaintances for medical advice.

Other medical personnel absolutely know the medical field in general better than those without any medical background.

But if you have a condition that could be serious, or if you're not getting better, play it safe and see a doctor (or a reliable mid-level practitioner such as a nurse practitioner or a physician assistant).

• Please write down, and keep a record of, any injections or vaccines you're given, whether you're at your doctor's office, a clinic, or an emergency room.

This information is so easy for you to get when you're there, and yet so hard to get once you leave.

And it can be so important for your short-term and long-term care to know exactly what injections you were given.

So when you're at the front desk checking out, just ask what medication—name and dosage—you were given. Your future doctors will be so pleased that they don't have to guess, make phone calls, or fill out forms to get this information.

Always trust your intuition

• Always trust your intuition when encountering problems with your body and interfacing with the healthcare system.

You care the most and know your loved one the best. Listen to your intuition and follow it.

Don't be talked out of it—it could save your loved one's life someday.

Intuition: fact or fiction?

• The belief in "intuition" has gone in and out of favor throughout history. For the first half of the 20th century, e.g., intuition was mostly seen and counted on as a helpful and protective part of being human. With the advent of great strides in medical and scientific knowledge, however, especially in the latter quarter of the 20th century, "intuition" became suspect. It just wasn't "scientific enough." Where's your data? How can you prove what you're feeling has any basis in truth or fact?

Doctors, probably because of their super-scientific training, became especially short on patience with those who might say something like "but I just feel it's something different" or "something just isn't right" or "but I know my child (or brother, or husband, or father) and this isn't normal *for him*."

But others didn't abandon this "unscientific" belief, and feel like it's worked well for them—consider, e.g., the belief in "a mother's intuition."

Pat Croskerry, M.D., Ph.D., has not abandoned the thought that we have instincts that are unexplainable scientifically. He writes in a 2005 article about decision-making and how we think:

> "Instincts, in the ethological sense, are hard-wired chunks of inherited behavior, and while it is readily accepted that animals have such inherited behavior patterns, *there is a palpable reluctance to accept the same of humans.*
>
> Yet, there are persuasive arguments that we may be hard-wired to respond to certain features of our environment as well as to processing information in predictable ways."*

So, if your doctor dismisses your "feeling" or "intuition"—your *instinct* that says something's not right—then he might gain some insight by reading this article by Dr. Croskerry.

And in the meantime, you keep listening and responding to your own intuition about yourself and your loved ones.

*Croskerry, Pat. “The Theory and Practice of Clinical Decision-Making.” *Canadian Journal of Anesthesia* 52(6) (2005): R1-R8, *italics added*.

Chapter Four

Your Responsibility As an Inpatient

"A general lack of information on and awareness of errors in health care by purchasers and consumers makes it impossible for them to demand better care."*

*Institute of Medicine. *To Err Is Human: Building a Safer Health System.* Linda T. Kohn, Janet M. Corrigan, and Molla S. Donaldson, eds. Washington, D.C.: National Academy Press, 2000, p. 21.

Basically, there are two separate medical scenarios: being an "out-patient"—being treated by a doctor when *not* in a hospital, and being an "inpatient"—being treated by a doctor while *in* a hospital.

This chapter is advice to use when you are an inpatient.

An inpatient is in a very precarious position

• Remember that almost 100,000 patients die in U.S. hospitals every year due to medical errors,[1] and that there are certain things you can *and should* do to help ensure that your loved one is not in that statistic.

The U.S. healthcare system is not a smooth-running machine—it is riddled with errors and lack of safety checks. You must step in as *the person most interested in keeping your loved one alive and in good health*, and gently and respectfully, but insistently, make certain that he gets the healthcare he needs.

"One in 10 patients admitted to the hospital will suffer an adverse event as a result of their medical treatment. A reduction in adverse events could happen if patients could be engaged successfully in monitoring their care."*

"A true paradox exists in American hospital medicine: although we have more medical knowledge and better technology, there is evidence that inpatient medical care is becoming more disjointed and health care providers are experiencing increasing degrees of disconnection from their patients."†

*Davis, R.E., M. Koutantji, and C.A. Vincent. "How Willing Are Patients to Question Healthcare Staff on Issues Related to the Quality and Safety of their Healthcare? An Exploratory Study." *Quality and Safety in Healthcare* 17 (2008): 90-96.

†Phillips, Robert A., and Julia D. Andrieni. Editorial: "Translational Patient Care: A New Model for Inpatient Care in the 21st Century." *Archives of Internal Medicine* 167(19) (2007): 2025-2026.

The most important safeguard for the hospitalized patient—*you*

• *Absolutely the most important thing for an inpatient:* keep a close relative or a friend sitting with the patient 24/7.

When people aren't feeling well, they are not good advocates for themselves. They need someone there with them who can help.

It wasn't this way years ago, but in our modern hospital culture, doctors spend only a couple minutes a day in the room with the patient; nurses are busy with medication-giving, IV changing, and other organizing and administrative duties; nursing assistants are busy getting vital signs and running for supplies; and the ward clerk is busy answering the phone and arranging for tests to get done and getting the patient transferred to the right place at the right time.

There is absolutely no one presently at the hospital who actually *cares* for your loved one, like we remember that nurses used to do. The loved ones of the patient *must fill in that gap*, or the patient runs the risk of being a victim of our current busy, busy, busy healthcare system.[1, 10]

You need to be there to help make sure that everything goes right. From sending the wrong patient down for a procedure, to giving the wrong medications, hospitals are fraught with errors, and if the patient has someone by his side to just make sure that the only things that are happening to him are the ones that have been ordered, then that patient has a tremendous advantage in not becoming a medical error statistic.

The Joint Commission is an organization that evaluates and accredits hospitals, and holds them to certain standards. It recognizes the problems in getting safe medical care, and has launched a national campaign to urge patients to take a more pro-active role in monitoring their hospital care. Here is one of the key features of this campaign.

"Ask a trusted family member or friend to be your advocate. Ask this person to stay with you, *even overnight*, when you are hospitalized. You will be able to rest better. Your advocate can help make sure you get the right medicines and treatments."*

If you're still on the fence on this issue, as in "but I'll be in the way," or "the nurses are there to take care of him"—then don't get in the way, and realize that hospital nurses have too many demands on their time to spend any significant time at your loved one's bedside watching over him.

Read Endnote 1 about medical errors in hospitals being the *6th leading cause of death.* Read Endnote 10 about how often errors happen in the hospital.

And don't leave your loved one alone in the hospital *unless* he has a minor, stable condition. And even then, check on him frequently.

> "There is an emerging body of opinion in the international literature that *patients and their families/nominated carers have an important role to play in monitoring and improving patient safety in health care settings*. Underpinning this view is a growing appreciation of the unique relationship that exists between patients and their families, and their collective capacity to provide continuous vigilance over both the patient's health condition and the care that is given. It is also being increasingly recognized that, unlike others who come and go, patients and their families are often situated as 'privileged witnesses of events ... who observe almost the whole process of care'. *As well as this, during the trajectory of their health care experience, patients often become 'experts' in their own illnesses and care* and, as has been shown, can become very adept at recognizing and rescuing *errors* (e.g., wrong drug administration), *near misses* (e.g., tests performed on the wrong patient) and *adverse events* (e.g., unanticipated adverse reactions to medications; post-surgical complications) that may not otherwise be captured by a hospital's incident reporting system or patient case notes. This has led some commentators to suggest that many patients and families are well positioned (during and shortly after a hospital stay) to be a 'potentially useful source of information that could inform clinical care and guide improvement initiatives.'"†

*The Joint Commission. "Speak Up™ Program." www.jointcommission.org/NR/rdonlyres/484AD48F-C464-4B5B-8D70-AA79179B3970/0/Speakup.pdf, *accessed* November 15, 2008, *italics added*. "These efforts to increase patient awareness and involvement are also supported by the Centers for Medicare & Medicaid Services."

†Johnstone, Megan-Jane, and Olga Kanitsaki. "Engaging Patients as Safety Partners: Some Considerations for Ensuring a Culturally and Linguistically Appropriate Approach." *Health Policy* 2008, epub ahead of print, www.elsevier.com/locate/healthpol, *citing, respectively,* Koutantji, M., R. Davis, C. Vincent, and A. Coulter. "The Patient's Role in Patient Safety: Engaging Patients, Their Representatives, and Health Professionals." *Clinical Risk* 11 (2005): 99-104; *and* Weingart, S.N., O. Pagovich, and D.Z. Sands et al. "What Can Hospitalized Patients Tell Us about Adverse Events? Learning from Patient Reported Incidents." *Journal of General Internal Medicine* 20 (2005): 830-836; *italics added.*

The bedside advocate (the "*patient*-sitter")

• When a person is so sick that he's hospitalized, he really can't be the best advocate for himself, and careless things can happen when he's alone.

The person sitting with the patient can be a family member, a close friend, or even someone you hire. But this essential position—ensuring the safety of your loved one—is not for the faint of heart.

We'll call this person the "bedside advocate" (also sometimes called the "patient advocate"), but as far as the hospital is concerned, just call yourself whatever feels comfortable. (For example, "I'm just here to help" or "I'm the patient's assistant.") Medical personnel may still get offended if they think you doubt that everything is under control.

One day, when all hospitals, doctors, nurses and other medical personnel *get it* that family members are necessary for the good health of the patient, then the job of the bedside advocate will become easier.

For now, some doctors and nurses still haven't accepted that the limitations placed on them by bureaucratic demands have left many patients in jeopardy, and so family members *must* step in to help.

But just ask any doctor or nurse. They know the medical system, and they wouldn't leave their loved ones alone either!

Staying with your hospitalized loved one is *more important* than almost anything you might need to do outside the hospital

• Understandably, the spouse or parent of a patient has a job, children or other responsibilities to take care of.

Nonetheless, your most *important* job at this time is to either stay at the hospital with your loved one, or find a trusted person who can.

Remember that your hospitalized loved one is at great risk because of the lack of checks and controls in the current healthcare system.[10] Use your time where you are most needed.

Ask any of the millions of people who have lost someone to a hospital error—they would *never* again leave their loved one without someone there.

The person sitting with the patient can be a family member, a close friend, or even someone you hire.

If you don't have a lot of people to help with the 24/7 schedule, then it would be best for the main advocate (a spouse or parent) to stay at the hospital as much as possible, and sleep there by the patient as well, in the chair provided, or bring a camp chair.

Hospitals often have less staff working at night, so don't believe for a second that when you go home your loved one will be well-taken care of.

The bedside advocate can usually doze in the chair at night and often during the day if he needs more sleep.

But please get some help for this 24-hour job if you can.

"Patient safety problems of many kinds occur during the course of providing health care. They include transfusion errors and adverse drug events; wrong-site surgery and surgical injuries; preventable suicides; restraint-related injuries or death; hospital-acquired or other treatment-related infections; and falls, burns, pressure ulcers, and mistaken identity."*

*Institute of Medicine. *To Err Is Human: Building a Safer Health System.* Linda T. Kohn, Janet M. Corrigan, and Molla S. Donaldson, eds. Washington, D.C.: National Academy Press, 2000, p. 35.

Patient must assert his need for the bedside advocate

• Let your loved one (the patient) know that it is important that the bedside advocate be there and that the patient needs to assert his need for that person if asked by the nurses or doctors.

It is very important for the patient to follow these instructions.

For example, if the doctor or nurse asks the bedside advocate to leave the room, the patient needs to say, "I want him to stay—he promised he wouldn't leave me."

Have a letter signed by the patient stating the patient's desire for his own 24/7 assistant or bedside advocate. Make sure the letter says that the patient wants all of his medical information given to his bedside advocate. Tape it to the wall, so that the hospital staff can see it.

The Joint Commission (that hospitals recognize as an authority) advises you to do the following:

"Ask a family member or friend to be your advocate (advisor or supporter).

- Find out if there is a form you need to fill out to name your personal representative, also called an advocate. [Or write one yourself.]
- Your advocate can ask questions that you may not think about when you are stressed.
- Ask this person to stay with you, *even overnight*, when you are hospitalized. You will be able to rest better. Your advocate can help make sure you get the right medicines and treatments.
- Your advocate can also help remember answers to questions you have asked. He or she can speak up for you when you cannot speak up for yourself."*

"These efforts to increase patient awareness and involvement are also supported by the Centers for Medicare & Medicaid Services."*

*The Joint Commission. "Speak Up™ Program." www.jointcommission.org/GeneralPublic/Speak+Up/about_speakup.htm, *accessed* November 15, 2008, *italics added*; and www.

jointcommission.org/NR/rdonlyres/58A5230D-3E58-48D8-8114-C95AF53ECA27/0/Speak up_ Rights.pdf, *accessed* November 15, 2008.

General info for the bedside advocate

• In order to "earn" your place as part of the team, the bedside advocate must be prepared to act calmly, respectfully, considerately and helpfully. Once doctors and nurses see that most advocates are acting this way, then we will be welcomed.

▪ *Stay out of the way.* The bedside advocate should be "background"—not in the foreground.

▪ *Don't get into confrontations with doctors or nurses.* The bedside advocate should not get into confrontations with doctors or nurses.

If you feel that there are problems you can't surmount by talking with the medical personnel right there, then ask for the charge nurse (also sometimes called the nursing supervisor), the hospital's patient advocate, the hospital administrator, or anyone in Risk Management.

Don't get into anger or blaming—just assert what you need from whom.

▪ *Be helpful.* The bedside advocate should be helpful to the nurses and personnel. If you can get your loved one what he needs, then do so. Be a positive influence in the care of the patient and take over any minor tasks that you can to help out the nursing staff.

Don't intervene in medical duties though, unless invited by the nursing staff, or if you get to know them well enough to ask them to let you help.

Leave the machines completely alone so that the medical personnel don't feel like you're a threat to good care.

▪ *Keep the noise level and number of visitors at any one time down.* Definitely be respectful and keep the noise level and the number of visitors down if you are sharing a room with another patient. Even if you have a private room, make sure that you are not making noise and disturbances with visitors that carry into the hall and can affect other patients and their families. (Even if your loved one is recovering well, there might be a family next door that is facing more somber news.)

▪ *Clear the way for hospital personnel to work.* Train family and friends to clear out of the way as soon as any hospital personnel come into the room. (Back away from the bed and out of the way.) If the nurse or doctor asks for everyone to leave the room, the bedside advocate should help to get everyone to leave right away, and then place herself in a corner of the room, out of the way.

In this way, the hospital personnel will come to appreciate your place there, and note your helpfulness.

▪ *Be sensitive that the medical personnel have a lot (too much!) to do.* Don't bother them with questions you don't need answered. Let them do their jobs, and don't take up their time with "I'm just curious" questions.

You can get a friend to do some Internet searching and bring you some information on things you're curious about while you're in the hospital with your loved one, instead of taking up precious time from the professionals. (And you'll really get better information as well, because it won't be from someone who's rushed and just wants to get on to her or his next task.)

Keep a hospital journal

• Now bedside advocate, you're going to have to be brave and assertive. Not aggressive or antagonistic, but assertive.

In order to help protect your loved one from undesirable medical errors, you're going to have to keep a journal of everything that happens to your loved one. This will include checking to make sure he gets the medications he needs and the procedures that are ordered (and *only* those).

I know you don't want to do this. I know it makes you feel uncomfortable. I know you think it's not your job.

If you think you want to avoid having to do this, then read Endnotes 1 and 4 about medical errors and misdiagnosed and mismanaged healthcare. Read Endnote 10 about how often errors happen in the hospital.

Read these statements from the Institute of Medicine:

> "Patient partnering [having patients involved in their medicines and treatments] is not a substitute for nursing responsibility to give the proper medication properly or for physicians to inform their patients, *but because no one is perfect*, it provides an opportunity to intercept the rare but predictable error."*
>
> "They [patients] should be encouraged to notify their doctors or staff of discrepancies in medication administration or the occurrence of side effects. If they are encouraged to take this responsibility, *they can be a final 'fail-safe' step*."*

If you feel like your patient is up to it, then give him the journal and tell him to go at it. But in my experience, most hospitalized patients are too sick to do this on their own. They need to spend all their time resting and getting well. So that leaves *you* to be the "final 'fail-safe' step."*

Have a journal at the bedside, and have each bedside advocate use the journal—write down the date, what medications the patient takes at what time, when thc doctors come in, the vital signs of the patient, and any treatments that are given. Also register the time when the patient or family calls for assistance, and the time it is given.

An example of this journal is at www.CautiousPatient.org for you to download.

If asked what you are doing, and you *will* be asked by everybody, explain that you are "keeping a log (or journal) of John's hospital experience."

Or you can say "I'm just here to assist John in any way I can since he's sick and can't always do everything for himself."

(Or you could let them know that you're doing what the patient has asked you to do; or that the Institute of Medicine recommends that the patient be the final checkpoint to catch any medication errors; or that the Joint Commission has asked the patient to be more involved in his care, and should have an advocate to help.)

When you have a log of the medicines given, ask the doctor when he visits to look over the list and see that it's right. Note in the journal that the doctor looked it over and said it was correct.

Some hospitals are so progressive now that they will even give you a copy of the medication sheet so that you can see what *should* be given. Ask if that's the case where you are.

The sad but true fact about hospital medications is that up to one of every five medications is given incorrectly.[10] Another fact is that although doctors order the medicine, they don't check to see how, when or even *if* it is given.

Many times nurses still give a medicine days after it was discontinued. There's just no way the "system" can catch that error easily. And sometimes the patient doesn't get the medicine that the doctor ordered, or doesn't get it for the proper length of time.

Family members *must* be the final check on the medication, and on making sure that your loved one is getting the procedures that are ordered, and *only* the procedures that are ordered.

So do your loved one a favor, and be this important, final checkpoint for him.

And to help you know what you should do, and give you some extra support, go to the Joint Commission's website at www.jointcommission.org, and pay special attention to their Speak Up Initiatives. A few of their pointers have been included in Endnote 10.

"Of all medical errors, medication errors are one of the most common ... They account for 19% to 20% of all adverse events. Of all hospitalized patients, 2.43% develop a clinically important adverse drug event during their hospitalization."[†]

"Providing the proper drug therapy to a hospitalized patient involves several steps and multiple individuals; a mistake at any point in the process ... may lead to a significant error."[‡]

*Institute of Medicine. *To Err Is Human: Building a Safer Health System.* Linda T. Kohn, Janet M. Corrigan, and Molla S. Donaldson, eds. Washington, D.C.: National Academy Press, 2000, p. 196, *italics added.*

†Lehmann, Christoph U., and George R. Kim. "Prevention of Medication Errors." *Clinics in Perinatology* 32 (2005): 107-123.

‡Taylor, James A., Lori A. Loan, Judy Kamara, Susan Blackburn, and Donna Whitney. "Medication Administration Variances before and after Implementation of Computerized Physician Order Entry in a Neonatal Intensive Care Unit." *Pediatrics* 121(1) (2008): 123-128.

Getting the information you need for the hospital journal

• Now, this could be a very easy thing to do, but it also could be tough, depending on whom you're dealing with.

You'll probably have a nurse who is pleasant and just gives you the information you ask. More and more nurses are doing this, as they have been informed that it is a good idea for the patient to know about and be involved in his care.

But occasionally, nursing personnel can be curt or brusque with you for asking questions about what medicines are being given, or what the vital signs are, as if it is some sort of classified information. In the unlikely event that this happens, just be calm and say that you're just trying to keep a record, and you'd appreciate them giving you that information. Simple human courtesy should require the nurse to answer reasonable questions.

If another strategy is needed, you might need to remind the nurse (or whomever) that you know that one of the Joint Commission's patient safety goals for hospitals (Goal #13) is to "encourage patients' active involvement in their own care as a patient safety strategy,"* and that you're just helping the patient to be involved in his care. Nurses and other hospital personnel are pretty well-acquainted with rules that the Joint Commission wants them to follow, because the Joint Commission accredits the hospitals.

That should be all you need to do to get the information you need.

On very rare occasions when the nurse is not cooperative, you might have to resort to the following strategies.

If they're not giving you the information you ask for, you might need to follow them into the hall with your journal, and ask them to call their nursing supervisor or charge nurse to come and give you the information if they are unable to.

Speak calmly and respectfully. Stay with her until she calls the nursing supervisor or gives you the information you're seeking; alternatively, ask the ward clerk (the non-medical person who sits at the nursing station who answers the phone) to call the charge nurse, or pick up the hospital phone yourself and ask the operator to page the charge nurse to come to your room.

If you run into a brick wall, request that they call the doctor if they think they need to get permission to give you this information. Have handy the letter that the patient has signed asking that the bedside advocate be given all of the patient's medical information.

If you need to, call the hospital's patient advocate, the hospital administrator or anyone in Risk Management. You might have to assert the patient's HIPAA rights. HIPAA (pronounced "hip'-uh") is a federal law that gives the patient a right to his medical information. You can quote the Joint Commission on your responsibility to speak up when you want answers (see Speak Up campaign in Endnote 10).

Again, most nurses today are used to patients and their advocates asking a lot of questions, and you'll probably not run into a problem. But if you do, just stay calm, and be prepared.

*Joint Commission. "2008 National Patient Safety Goals: Critical Access Hospital Program." www.jointcommission.org/PatientSafety/NationalPatientSafetyGoals/08_cah_npsgs.htm, *accessed* November 30, 2008.

Go with your loved one when he leaves his room

• If your patient is sent to x-ray or another part of the hospital for a test or procedure, *go with him*. "Transportation" at the hospital typically sends an orderly to take your loved one to these places, but oftentimes your loved one is then set on the side of a hall, either coming or going, and doesn't have anyone to help him out.

Medical personnel will assure you that you won't be needed, *and* aren't wanted, but just be respectful and patient, and say that you'll just walk with them (the orderly and the bed) and wait for your loved one during the test. You'll stay out of their way.

Be a respectful advocate for your loved one—if the wait seems long, check with someone. You will be the "legs" that go to find out what is going on for them or ask for something they need.

If they are going into a room for some tests, you may not be allowed in that room, and that is okay. Tell everyone you'll just be waiting outside until they come out. Ask how long the test should take, and then take action (ask somebody what's going on) if the time gets longer than expected.

Medical errors have been noted to be frequent when patients are in transition from one place to another.

Be there for your loved one.

Be kind to the nurses

• There may possibly be no harder job than that of a hospital nurse.

Nurses are there to assess you and decide what your nursing needs are, and then to formulate goals and plans based on those needs; they implement those plans; and then they continually re-evaluate how those plans are working to help you get well and stay free from complications while in the hospital,

in addition to

following doctor's orders—preparing and giving regular medications, inserting IVs or NG tubes, taking vital signs, and supervising your mobility status,

as well as

watching for changes in your clinical condition, and calling for help if they believe that things are changing in your condition and you now need to be re-assessed by the doctor,

plus

documenting charts, supervising aides, searching for supplies, and giving medications as needed to help you with pain or unpleasant symptoms.

Nurses have to keep a large amount of information about each patient they're responsible for *in their heads*, as they physically shift between different patients, while also answering questions from nursing aides or assistants about other patients.

And studies show that RNs are frequently interrupted in their duties, making everything that much harder.

One of the worst things of all is that most states don't have a legislated nurse to patient ratio. That is, each hospital on any particular day can assign whatever number of patients that they want to assign to the care of an RN. And even if the nurse knows that she doesn't have time to do the right care for that number of patients—there's *nothing* she can do about it except do the best she can, in the face of unrealistic demands.

So, *your* very serious problem, when your loved one is in the hospital, is that you don't know whether the nurse to patient ratio that includes your loved one is adequate or not. And if it's adequate during the day, then it may not be during the night, or during another shift.

Also, some hospitals *require* nurses to take on extra shifts when they are short on personnel, even though research has adamantly shown that after twelve hours on the job, the quality of their work suffers. So you don't know if you have a tired nurse either.

Research also has shown that a higher RN to patient ratio is safer for patients. (You want a higher ratio. A higher ratio means that one nurse takes care of fewer patients.)

So, nurses have a noble calling, but in real life, they have really tough jobs—lots of serious responsibilities, but often with working hours and conditions where they feel they can't always do right by the patient, except to try to work faster and faster.

All this, plus they have to deal with doctors. (A survey found that over 20% of hospital nurses leave their jobs because of issues over the way doctors treat them.)

So what can you do?

Here are a few suggestions:

▪ 1. Be there 24/7 for your loved one, so that *your* loved one isn't the one hitting the call button for an hour before he can get a bedpan.

▪ 2. Be there 24/7 for your loved one so that you can go out and find a nurse yourself if you see something wrong.

▪ 3. Be there for your elderly loved one at night so he doesn't have to be tied to the bedrails.

Elderly patients often get disoriented in the hospital at night, and the nurses have to put them into "restraints" in order to keep them from pulling out their tubes or trying to get out of bed.

Even if your loved one has to be in restraints, at least you'll be there to scratch his nose, give him a sip or water and comfort him.

▪ 4. Be there for the nurses. When you first see a nurse who's working with your loved one, mention that you know that nurses are overworked, and ask her how you might be of assistance to *her* in helping the patient. Watch what she's doing, and if you think it's appropriate, ask if you can take over that chore, to save her some time.

You might also ask each day when you see your assigned nurse of that day, "What can I do on *your shift today* that would give you more time and make a positive contribution to the patients on this ward?" The nurse might be able to give you some ideas, and at least she would know your heart is in the right place.

▪ 5. Don't complain about the little things. Take care of the little things yourself.

▪ 6. Be sure to give them any nice comments. They are so overworked and under-appreciated.

▪ 7. If public policy is your thing, support nurses in their efforts to get state legislatures to make sure that they don't have to take care of more patients than they can safely handle.

I mean, my child's kindergarten class had a teacher-student ratio of 1 to 22, and when 23 kids showed up to enroll, they were obligated by state law to split the class into two. So when it comes to nursing care and patient safety, why should we do less?

> "Responding to research confirming the link between nurse staffing and patient outcomes, 14 states have introduced legislation to limit patient-to-nurse ratios ... Eight patients per nurse was the least expensive ratio but was associated with the highest patient mortality. Decreasing the number of patients per nurse improved mortality ... As a patient safety intervention, patient-to-nurse ratios of 4:1 are reasonably cost-effective and in the range of other commonly accepted [patient safety] interventions."*

"Many RNs believe that state or federal government regulations are the only mechanism that can raise nurse staffing levels to a point where they are adequate to meet patient needs."[†]

*Rothberg, Michael B., Ivo Abraham, Peter K. Lindenauer, and David N. Rose. "Improving Nurse-to-Patient Staffing Ratios As a Cost-Effective Safety Intervention." *Medical Care* 43(8) (2005): 785-791.

†Litvak, Eugene, Peter I. Buerhaus, Frank Davidoff, Michael C. Long, Michael L. McManus, and Donald M. Berwick. "Managing Unnecessary Variability in Patient Demand to Reduce Nursing Stress and Improve Patient Safety." *Joint Commission Journal on Quality and Patient Safety* 31(6) (2005): 330-338.

Hospital nurses are also patient advocates: they help prevent infections, medication errors, medical complications and deaths

• Not to be taken lightly is the role that nurses play in your safe recovery while in the hospital.[11]

But most hospital nurses feel that they are overwhelmed by the amount of work assigned to them, and feel that they can't keep patients safe under their present working conditions.[11]

That's another reason why you have to be there to help the nurses protect your loved one.

And good nurses will understand the need for you to be there—trust me, they wouldn't leave *their* loved ones in the hospital alone!

"The evidence indicates that inadequate nurse staffing leads to adverse patient outcomes ... The AHRQ reports that a vast amount of research has shown a relationship between lower nurse staffing and higher rates of adverse patient outcome ... Shock, cardiac arrest, UTIs [bladder infections], and pneumonia were all negative outcomes *associated with low nurse staffing levels*."*

"*Nurses have a critical patient advocacy role*: the total number of errors would be greater if nurses did not intercept 86% of all potential errors that could result in patient harm."†

*Garrett, Connie. "The Effect of Nurse Staffing Patterns on Medical Errors and Nurse Burnout." *AORN Journal* 87(6) (2008): 1191-1204, *italics added.*

†Hughes, Ronda G., and Carolyn M. Clancy. "Working Conditions That Support Patient Safety." *Journal of Nursing Care Quality* 20(4) (2005): 289-292, *italics added.*

What if the doctor asks you to leave the room?

• Doctors and nurses ask you to leave the room out of habit—it's just always been done that way.

It's like thirty years ago, husbands and family members were kept out of the delivery rooms, and now that's a really outdated idea.

Telling family members to wait in the waiting room or limiting the time they can watch over their critically-ill loved one is another outdated idea.

If a doctor asks you to wait outside, just say calmly yet confidently, "I'm going to stay out of your way, but I need to be here." Then back away from the patient to the side of the room where you *are* out of the way.

If they ask again, just respectfully say that you promised the patient you wouldn't leave him, and you won't interfere. Stay respectful and non-threatening.

Sometimes, the patient may need to help by speaking up; for example, "I need my sister to stay." Most doctors will not oppose the patient's wishes.

But if you come across a particularly difficult doctor, you may need to talk with the hospital's patient advocate, or the hospital administrator.

Sometimes it might be a good idea to quietly sit down in the corner, and say "I'll just stay over here." This might be helpful because doctors and nurses often justify their asking you to leave by saying that you're in the way or that you are going to faint and fall down, and they don't want to have to deal with "another" patient.

Do what you need to do to stay and be an advocate for your loved one.

Critically important advice: don't allow doctors or nurses to ignore your concerns

• Always trust your intuition and make sure your health providers are listening. You know your loved one better than anyone else.

If you can't get your doctor or nurse to listen and act on your concerns, then contact the hospital's patient advocate. Many hospitals now have them, and they are vital to patient safety. If one isn't handy, ask for the charge nurse, the hospital administrator, or anyone in Risk Management.

Over and over again, loved ones who have lost someone to medical error relate that they knew something was wrong, but they weren't listened to or taken seriously.

Don't let this happen to you.

But if you can't get your doctor's or nurse's attention ...

If the patient's condition is deteriorating...

• If your loved one is in the hospital, he's getting worse, you're very worried that adequate attention is not being paid to it, and you believe it to be critical, then call for a "rapid response team." These teams have been developed for those situations where a patient's condition is deteriorating, the reason is unknown, and steps are not being taken to correct the problem.[12]

Rapid response teams have been put into play to come at a moment's notice and completely re-assess a patient who is getting worse without apparent reason. They bring immediate attention and a fresh perspective as they completely re-assess the patient.

They can literally be lifesaving.

If there is no rapid response team at your hospital, then call your doctor and insist that a physician come right away to re-assess the patient. If the doctor doesn't do so, then call the charge nurse, the hospital's patient advocate, the hospital administrator, or anyone in Risk Management.

You can also keep an eye on your loved one following some of the same criteria that are used to identify patients who have become unstable and need to be rapidly re-evaluated.

Watch for these warning signs in your loved one:

- ***Pulse*** less than 40 or greater than 130 beats per minute;
- ***Systolic blood pressure (BP)*** less than 90 (systolic BP is the first and higher of the two numbers—e.g., if BP is 120/80, then 120 is the systolic blood pressure);
- ***Breaths*** (respirations) less than 8 or more than 24 per minute;
- ***Seizure*** (convulsion) activity of any kind;
- ***Acute change in mental status*** (e.g., a person who is normally conscious and aware becoming delirious, confused, or "out-of-it").*

If these signs come and persist, then let the nurse know and get medical attention for your loved one immediately.

The following describes the implementation of some rapid response teams in the last several years:

"Community Health Network in Indianapolis has launched a new patient safety initiative, Call FIRST (Family-Initiated Rapid Screening Team), in all five of its hospitals. As part of the program, patients and their families are encouraged to make a phone call when there is a change in the patient's condition and they feel their concerns are not being addressed. A designated internal phone line has been established for the program at each facility. When the number is called, a nursing supervisor or consult nurse will provide help within 15 minutes at the bedside to evaluate and stabilize the situation ... The program is based on the 'Condition H' program started by the University of Pittsburgh Medical Center in 2005 ... 'There are a number of situations in which the program can prove beneficial,' says Wilson [vice president of nursing at Community Hospital North]. 'For example, there could be a case of a woman who has been with her husband for 20 years and knows he is not acting normal,' she says. 'The family members might recognize something that we don't.' Because of this added level of communication, she adds, 'We feel family involvement will increase patient safety.'"†

*Offner, Patrick J., Joseph Heit, and Robin Roberts. "Implementation of a Rapid Response Team Decreases Cardiac Arrest Outside of the Intensive Care Unit." *Journal of Trauma* 62(5) (2007): 1223-1228.

†Healthcare Benchmarks and Quality Improvement. "Program Increases Patient, Family Involvement: Patient Safety Initiative Honors NSPG [National Patient Safety Goals, recommended by Joint Commission]." *Healthcare Benchmarks and Quality Improvement* 14(12) (2007): 139-141.
See also Joint Commission's 2009 National Patient Safety Goals at www.jointcommission.org/patientsafety/nationalpatientsafetygoals.

Beware of the "one-disease-per-patient-limit"

• This concept is a little difficult to explain, but it occurs frequently, and you must understand it to get the care that you need and avoid disastrous consequences.

There's a sort of "tunnel-vision" that many, many doctors engage in when they see you as a patient. They focus on what you've told them to start with, they make an assessment, and then they don't re-assess you when further symptoms develop—they just assign those additional symptoms to the diagnosis that they decided on in the first place.

And if your new symptoms are the result of a new disease, and it's a life-threatening one, then you're in trouble if it goes undiagnosed.[4]

For example, if you're in the hospital after surgery, then the doctor's "perception" of you is that you're in the "post-surgical recovery stage." Then, when you report any symptoms, he tends to automatically assign them to the "post-surgical recovery process."

Where you get into trouble is when your new symptom is actually the presentation of a new and serious illness, but your doctor isn't thinking outside of his original perception. And if your new problem is serious, undiagnosed and untreated, the consequences can be deadly.

Imagine you entered the hospital with a certain condition like a kidney stone, and then find yourself with chest pain. If that had been your presenting symptom, your doctor would have done everything necessary to rule out a heart attack—but since you're in the hospital with a kidney stone, your doctor hears "pain" and everything else just isn't clicking because you've been assigned "kidney stone" in his mind, and he's not thinking that something *else* might be going on.

Here's where you have to listen to your body, your doctor *and* trust your intuition. If everything just doesn't seem to make sense, and if things aren't getting better, then do what you have to do to get your doctor to re-assess you.

You might say this to your doctor: "I know you're saying that [*this new symptom*] is a result of [*your already diagnosed illness*], but something just doesn't feel right to me, and I want you to re-assess me, just focusing on what else this new symptom could be."

And if your doctor isn't willing to do that, then insist that he call in a consultant who will.

And if you think the situation is urgent, then call for a rapid response team.

"Once a diagnosis has been established, it is often used to explain all newly occurring symptoms *without necessarily considering that another underlying disease might be present.*"*

*Kirch, Wilhelm, and Christine Schafii. "Misdiagnosis at a University Hospital in 4 Medical Eras: Report on 400 Cases." *Medicine* 75(1) (1996): 29-40, *italics added.*

Don't rely on nurses for diagnoses

• Sometimes you might experience a frightening, new, and disturbing symptom while you're in the hospital, and you'll call the nurse in to tell her about it. She should take your information, check your vital signs, and then call your doctor about the new development.

But sometimes a nurse will listen to you and then come up with her own diagnosis of what's wrong, and give you a version of what she thinks, and then go about her way.

If we're talking about something minor that's not causing you much discomfort, then you're probably okay, and you can wait until the doctor is making rounds.

But if your new symptom remains disturbing or painful, then you might be in danger from a complication or new illness. And then the nurse's failure to notify the doctor about the problem could be dangerous.

Nurses usually know when they can comment confidently and when they should call the doctor. But occasionally, several things can get in the way of the nurse's best judgment: too much to do/too many patients to care for; double-shifts or tiredness; inexperience; or dreading to call the doctor (more on this later).

So if a new symptom develops while you're in the hospital, and it's troubling and you feel it could be important, be respectfully insistent that a doctor be called to examine you.

If you can't get the nurse to call the doctor, then call for the charge nurse, the hospital's patient safety advocate, the hospital administrator, or anyone in the Risk Management Department.

And you can call for a rapid response team if it appears particularly urgent.

One note: specialty nurses, who have had special training on patients with a certain condition, are incredibly valuable to your safe care. These nurses have been trained to handle some analysis and decision-making on their own in their specialty areas, so you can usually rely on their advice in the areas they're trained in.

You're usually in the best hospital situation possible when you have a nurse attending to you who has been specially trained about patients with your particular condition, *and* who has a good teamwork relationship with your doctor. (More about this later.)

Even so, if you feel uncomfortable with a nurse's handling of a new symptom, go ahead and listen to your intuition and ask for a doctor to re-assess your situation. As with any other healthcare worker, there may be times that fatigue, too many patients, or some other factor may be interfering with her best judgment. Follow your instinct.

It's not you: some doctors are jerks

• To be kinder, let's just say that some doctors should have been raised better. Some are flippant, arrogant, sarcastic, thoughtless, insensitive, and antagonistic.

Most doctors are *not* like this; but medicine certainly seems to have its fair share of high-handed, short-tempered, self-important individuals—individuals who don't obey the rules of common courtesy and throw tantrums like two-year-old children.

Who knows if they start out that way or develop it during their medical training, but if you can get away from a doctor like this, it's to your advantage.

Why? Because research shows that hospitalized patients with that kind of doctor may be at extra risk, because the communication between the doctors and nurses is so negatively affected by that doctor's behavior, that nurses don't want to have to deal with them, and so they avoid calling that doctor, even though it may be warranted.[13]

Read Endnote 13 to learn more about how much damage these doctors do.

"Disruptive, intimidating, or abusive behavior may increase the likelihood of errors by leading nurses, residents, or colleagues to avoid the disruptive physician, to hesitate to ask for help or clarification of orders, and to hesitate to make suggestions about patient care."*

"They're out there ... browbeating nurses and pharmacists, dressing down hapless staff, belittling patients to their faces, swearing at the tops of their voices, muttering ominous threats, dripping sarcasm and snide innuendo, slouching in late day after day, raging, sulking, hurling surgical instruments, blowing off appointments, sabotaging meetings, sneering at administrators ... oh yes, you name it, no matter how outrageous, one of them is pretty sure to have done it ... because ... they're out there: The Problem Docs."†

And don't believe for a moment that their attitude is due to their "superior talent" or "high standards." It's only on TV that this sort of arrogant, sarcastic individual is actually the smartest doc in the group—there it makes for good comedy and drama.

In real life, it means that that doc just has personality problems, and likes to throw his weight around like a wrecking ball. And unfortunately his patients suffer the most.

It's best to avoid one of these doctors for the sake of your health, as well as on general principle.

*Leape, Lucian L., and John A. Fromson. "Problem Doctors: Is There a System-Level Solution?" *Annals of Internal Medicine* 114(2) (2006): 107-115.

†Weber, David O. "Poll Results: Doctors' Disruptive Behavior Disturbs Physician Leaders." *Physician Executive* 2004 (September-October): 6-14.

Prevent hospital infections

• *Hospital-acquired infections are deadly.*[14] Hospital-acquired infections in U.S. hospitals occur 1.7 million times a year, and 99,000 patients *die* each year from those infections.*

The bedside advocate is the patient's best shield against acquiring an infection.

Keep a bottle of gel hand sanitizer (like Purell) in the hospital room near you. When any nurses, doctors, other hospital staff or visitors come into the room, the bedside advocate should walk or lean toward them and help them take some into their palm.

Say "we're asking everyone who comes in to use this hand sanitizer." You could also tape a sign on the wall behind the patient's bed that says "Please use hand sanitizer when you come into the room," and you could point to that as you're offering the gel.

(This is not necessary if you see the medical personnel use a hand sanitizer as they come into the room—just make sure that you *see* them use the sanitizer.)

Here's an interesting suggestion given to me: ask the doctor if it would be a good idea if everyone washed their hands or used the gel when they come in. If he says "yes," then put up a sign that says "Always wash your hands or use gel—doctor's orders," and point to that sign when people come in the door. (And if he doesn't say "yes"—ask another doctor.)

If hospital personnel come into the room and then don a pair of gloves from a box at the door, then that's good enough in some cases (but not all, and the personnel *are* supposed to have washed their hands in addition to using gloves).

Be sure that the bedside advocate also uses the hand sanitizer, or washes his hands, *each time* he enters the room.

And never, *ever* pick up anything off the floor and continue to use it for the patient. Anything that hits the floor has to be sanitized immediately or trashed.

Most importantly, remember that the risky and potentially deadly infections that patients get while in the hospital *usually* start in a surgical wound, or where the patient has a break in his skin or a tube into his body, like where he has an IV catheter, or where he has a urine catheter. In fact, 32% of hospital-acquired infections are urinary tract infections; 22% are surgical wound infections; 15% are lung infections (pneumonia) (especially if your loved one is on a ventilator); and 14% are bloodstream infections (often from a contaminated IV site).*

So, be *especially vigilant* when anyone is about to touch a surgical wound, any open skin surface, or an IV site. *The people who touch those sites absolutely need to have freshly cleansed hands.*

Studies have shown that patients can often have their urine catheter taken out earlier than a doctor will remember to discontinue it (and when the urine catheter comes out, so does the chance of an infection to start that way).

Believe it or not, it's easy for a doctor to forget the urine catheter's there, because it's under the covers, and usually he's not focused on it. You can do the patient and his doctor a favor by reminding the doctor about it every day.

And the surgical wound—sometimes doctors actually forget to look at it! Keep your eye out, and make sure that a doctor looks at it at least once a day. And while he's looking at it, get a glimpse of it yourself, so you know what it looks like. Ask "is there any sign of infection?" while the doctor's looking at the wound, and you'll learn something about what wounds look like when they're healing fine and when they're infected.

Also look at the wound when the nurse uncovers it to put a new dressing on it.

Keep remembering the 99,000 people who die in the U.S. each year from hospital-acquired infections, and be vigilant about observing and protecting each place that your loved one might be vulnerable.*

And when your loved one leaves the hospital without having acquired one of these infections—celebrate! And congratulate all the nurses and the bedside advocates.

See Endnote 14 for specific handwashing recommendations.

Some doctors don't follow the rules for good hand hygiene, and need to be reminded to do so. Note Dr. Hoover's take on the stubbornness of many of his fellow surgeons in following patient safety protocols, including those regarding preventing infections:

"Surgeons have known since the exploits of Semmelweiss that hand washing is the most important single thing that they can do to control infections, but compliance decreases linearly from medical students to residents to attending surgeons. Senior surgeons continue to check wounds without wearing gloves and enter isolation rooms without donning gowns, gloves, and masks ... I have witnessed physicians entering the rooms of patients with methicillin-resistant *Staphylococcus aureus* [without proper precautions] when the rooms were clearly marked with every precaution sign in the repertoire and *all* were totally ignored by some of the most intelligent people on earth ... Complicating this is the fact that we have not yet empowered our other colleagues such as nurses, housekeeping staff, technicians, and dieticians to call us to task for violating protocol."[†]

"The people in the airline industry half-jokingly tell me that pilots are very diligent about reducing errors because, in every instance, they are the first ones to arrive at the scene of a fatal airline crash. Surgeons on the other hand may suffer mental anguish over deaths and complications in their patients, but they do not suffer bodily harm, and therein lies at least some of the explanation for their behavior."[†]

"Healthcare-associated infections are the most common complications affecting hospitalized patients, making infection control a priority for patient safety ... Low nurse staffing is associated with an increased infection risk, and a substantial proportion of all infections acquired in critical care could be prevented by maintaining staffing at a higher level ... Infections tend to occur only a few days after exposure to high workload ... This suggests that under the pressure of increased workload, healthcare workers do not comply with infection control measures, such as hand hygiene, due to time constraints ...However, the causal pathway linking low staffing level and infections is likely to be much more complex."‡

*CDC. http://www.cdc.gov/ncidod/dhqp/hai.html, *accessed* July 26, 2008.

†Hoover, Eddie L. Commentary: "Patient Safety and Surgeons: Why the Resistance?" *Archives of Surgery* 142(12) (2007): 1127-1128, *italics added.*

‡Hugonnet, Stephane, Jean-Claude Chevrolet, and Didier Pittet. "The Effect of Workload on Infection Risk in Critically Ill Patients." *Critical Care Medicine* 35(1) (2007): 76-81.

Every patient has the right to adequate pain control

• Pain that doesn't go away with routine pain medication is a warning sign. If the pain is a new symptom for your hospitalized loved one, or the pain has significantly increased, insist that a doctor come to re-assess the patient.

If your loved one is in pain, the hospital *must* respond. The Joint Commission, the organization that accredits hospitals, has mandated that hospital personnel *must* ask a patient about his level of pain, and if it is moderate or greater, *must* do something about it.

The bedside advocate needs to remind the patient that when the nurse comes in and asks "how are you today?"—that is not a social question, but that is actually the "pain" question. The patient must speak up and tell the nurse about his pain. Don't let the patient say "fine," which is a reflexive act when someone asks "how are you?"

The nurse will then write "no complaints" in her chart, because that is what she heard. Remind the patient to tell the nurse what is hurting or actually how he is physically feeling every time a nurse asks that question.

If the doctor says there's nothing more that can be done for the pain, then ask for a pain doctor to consult.

In an acute situation, if you're having no luck with getting the nurse to listen, then call for the charge nurse, the hospital's patient advocate, the hospital administrator, or anyone in Risk Management.

"In July 2000, the Joint Commission introduced a new objective to improve the quality of health care in the United States. Effective January 1, 2001, institutions [hospitals] wishing to be compliant became responsible for ensuring that pain would be assessed and managed in all patients. The Commission concluded that acute and chronic pain were major causes of patient dissatisfaction in our health care system, leading to slower recovery times, creating a burden for patients and their families, and increasing the costs to the health care system."*

But be careful and stay with your loved one on pain medicines, because with the increased use of pain medicines, hospitals have had more patients with "opioid over sedation adverse drug reactions," which means that patients were getting too much narcotic—more or less narcotic overdoses, which can be very dangerous.

But it was also found that over 90% of the narcotic overdose patients *were noted by nurses to have decreased consciousness* during the 12 hours prior to the narcotic overdose emergency.* Thus, if the nurses had acted to have the narcotic dose decreased when they noted the decreased level of consciousness in the patients, it is possible that many of these narcotic emergencies could have been averted.

SO, if you have a loved one in pain, make sure he gets what he needs as far as pain medication is concerned, but be there to make sure that he is either awake and alert, or sleeping but easily aroused by voice. If he becomes confused or cannot be aroused by voice, then alert the nurses right away.

That's just another reason why you need to be there. If the hospitalized patient is not complaining, the nurses really don't get to his side very often to assess him. You be there for him instead.

*Vila, Hector, Jr., Robert A. Smith, and Michael J. Augustyniak et al. "The Efficacy and Safety of Pain Management Before and After Implementation of Hospital-Wide Pain Management Standards: Is Patient Safety Compromised by Treatment Based Solely on Numerical Pain Ratings? *Anesthesia and Analgesia* 101 (2005): 474-480.

Protect your elderly loved one with a poster board

• Older patients who have had a sudden major illness onset often look very different than they were immediately before the illness; this can result in really inadequate treatment in the hospital.

That's because many doctors and nurses see the older, wrinkled patient who is now incoherent, comatose or just "out-of-it" from an acute illness, and may not realize that this person was very active until this illness event.

Since doctors and nurses see many patients who are really ill and unresponsive from Alzheimer's or people from nursing homes who are not "with it," they often assume that the elderly patient they're seeing now (*your* loved one) has been in that condition for some time, and they don't understand that this *particular* older patient was very active until this hospitalization.

So it's terribly important to let the staff know that your older loved one was really active before this present illness (if that was the case).

Get a poster board, or some sheets of paper, and write with a thick marker something like this: "This patient (my mother or Jane Doe) was playing bridge last week!" or "This patient (my dad or John Doe) was playing tennis last week!" or whatever the truth might be, and tape it to the wall and make sure the healthcare personnel see it.

If you have the opportunity, you can put up a good recent photo of the patient, and make sure you put the date of the photo in large, bold print so they're able to see that it was a recent one! Patients can look very different when they're seriously ill, and it will give the medical personnel a good perspective on your loved one that will translate to more appropriate medical care.

If you have a choice, use a hospital where visiting hours aren't limited, even in the ICU

• Try to keep your loved one from being admitted to a hospital where visiting hours are limited.

That can be particularly difficult for you if your loved one is in the intensive care unit (ICU); but many hospitals now allow a family member to stay overnight even in ICU rooms. Use these hospitals whenever possible.

Even in ICUs, some hospitals may reduce the nurse to patient ratio at night, and if your loved one's nurse gets tied up with another patient who is critically ill or crashing, then *your* loved one may not be able to get someone's attention—even in the ICU. Be there for him.

In addition, although one might think that the ICU is the best place for your loved one to get careful medical care, studies show that many errors occur there as well.

And the ICU is a very scary place for a critically ill patient. Be there to hold his hand. Just that one connection could be critical to his well-being.

"The complexity of intensive care and the medical conditions of patients admitted to intensive care units increases the likelihood of medical errors ... Medical errors appear to be common among patients requiring intensive care. Medical events resulting in an error can result in the need for additional life-sustaining treatments and, in some circumstances, can contribute to patient death."*

"One study found that the average ICU patient experiences 1.7 errors per day, nearly one-third of which are potentially life-threatening. Most involve communication problems."†

"Adverse events and serious errors involving critically ill patients were common and often potentially life-threatening. Although many types of errors were identified, failure to carry out intended treatment correctly was the leading category ... In general, medicine [the medical system] has focused more on determining what to do than on ensuring that plans are effectively executed."‡

"[In the ICU], sleep cycles of patients are disrupted by alarms or other disruptive sounds, by care providers taking vital signs or administering medications, and by the high and prolonged levels of lighting. It is estimated that between 12.5% and 38% of patients who arrive at the ICU alert and oriented show signs of dementia after extended stays."[§]

*Osmon, Stephen, Carolyn B. Harris, W. Claiborne Dunagan, Donna Prentice, Victoria J. Fraser, and Marin H. Kollef. "Reporting of Medical Errors: An Intensive Care Unit Experience." *Critical Care Medicine* 32(3) (2004): 727-733.

†Wachter, Robert M. "The End of the Beginning: Patient Safety Five Years After 'To Err Is Human.'" *Health Affairs* 2004 (July-December) (Suppl. Web Exclusives): W4-534 – W4-545, *citing* Donchin, Y., D. Gopher, and M Olin et al. "A Look into the Nature and Causes of Human Errors in the Intensive Care Unit." *Critical Care Medicine* 23(2) (1995): 294-300.

‡Rothschild, Jeffrey M., Christopher P. Landrigan, and John W. Cronin et al. "The Critical Care Safety Study: The Incidence and Nature of Adverse Events and Serious Medical Errors in Intensive Care." *Critical Care Medicine* 33(8) (2005): 1694-1700.

§Donchin, Yoel, and F. Jacob Seagull. "The Hostile Environment of the Intensive Care Unit." *Current Opinion in Critical Care* 8 (2002): 316-320.

When your back is against the wall ...

• If there are limited visiting hours where you are, and you don't have a choice about hospitals, you still must do whatever you need to do to stay with your hospitalized loved one.

Many detrimental things have happened to patients when they didn't have family members with them—ask the thousands of family members who have left the hospital thinking their loved one was in good hands, and then returned to find their loved one in serious danger or suffering unnecessarily.

Start with this: many times the posted visiting hours aren't strictly enforced, so just quietly and unobtrusively stay where you are when visiting hours are over. If someone comes in and says anything to you, just say that you're just going to stay and help a while longer.

If hospital personnel finally feel it necessary to "lay down the law," tell them about your promise to your loved one to stay with him. Show them the document that says your loved one wants a 24/7 bedside advocate when hospitalized. Tell them that you know the Joint Commission has advised patients to have a loved one stay with them 24 hours a day.

If they persist, respectfully ask that they contact the hospital's patient advocate for you to talk with before you leave, because you believe it would be a mistake to leave your loved one, since you'd promised you'd stay with him, and you just don't think it would be right to break that promise.

If told that the hospital's patient advocate is not available right then, ask for an emergency meeting with the hospital administrator, as this is a significant issue and a patient safety issue for your loved one. Make certain that you state your intention of just quietly watching over and being an extra hand to the patient if he needs it.

Make sure that the patient also stresses to the hospital personnel that they need the family member to stay.

Hospitals listen to patients a lot better than they listen to the families of patients. So if your loved one is conscious, make sure he stresses over and over again to the hospital personnel that he needs you to stay with him.

If needed, the patient could say "I can't sleep if he's not here," or "I get too scared and have to call the nurses too much."

Do what you need to, but do it quietly and respectfully. There are many power struggles in hospitals, and when there's a rule on the wall, and they don't like you, you won't win.

If you're in the hospital emergency room ...

• When you're a patient in the emergency room, you're neither an outpatient nor an inpatient, and in this "in-between" zone it is sometimes harder to get the help you might need. You're probably thinking I'm kidding, but many tragic situations have happened as a result of inattentive emergency room care.

Here's the most common problem: when you go to the emergency room, you might start out with some symptoms that would indicate a minor illness. Then, during the time that you're being "worked-up" and you're there waiting for lab or x-ray results, the symptoms get worse or you start to feel new symptoms that would now point to a much more serious illness.

It often takes a patient advocate (your friend or loved one) to get adequate attention for this new development. Although it's hard to believe, emergency room personnel may not re-assess your situation unless *absolutely pressed to do so*; and that inattention to new or worsening symptoms has caused devastating results for many patients.

This sounds unbelievable, but consider this true case: a patient went into the emergency room with a kidney stone, and *while there* had the onset of crushing chest pain (that would have caused him to call an ambulance if he were at home), but because he was in the emergency room with a different presenting symptom *the staff didn't feel like they needed to complete an additional work-up for the new symptom.* He ended up with major damage to his heart from an unrecognized heart attack, and his health was compromised for the rest of his life.

So, when you're in the emergency room, it's *very important* that you have someone stay with you at all times, just as if you were an inpatient.

Also, re-read the "Don't allow doctors or nurses to ignore your concerns" section, and follow those instructions in the emergency room as well.

If you're in the emergency room and you don't feel your concerns are being taken seriously, then respectfully ask the doctor to write your concerns into the chart, and ask the nurse to enter your concerns into the nurse's notes.

If you're getting pushback from both doctors and nurses, mention that you believe this is a *patient safety issue*, and you need to talk with the hospital's patient advocate or the hospital administrator immediately.

Also be aware that studies have found errors in diagnosis as being a problem in emergency rooms.

In a 2005 study, Daudelin et al. found that about 26,000 patients are sent home annually from U.S. emergency rooms with a missed diagnosis of heart attack/unstable heart condition, which *nearly doubled the death rate for those patients.**

"Diagnostic errors in the emergency department (ED) are an important patient safety concern .... A total of 79 claims (65%) involved missed ED diagnoses that harmed patients. Forty-eight percent of these missed diagnoses were associated with serious harm, and 39% *resulted in death*."†

"The specialties with the largest proportion of highly preventable adverse events are general medicine ... and emergency medicine. Negligent errors in emergency and urgent care are usually due to delayed or incorrect diagnoses."‡

"'By directly involving patients in their own care, and encouraging them to inform their providers of any signs of errors, the level of safety can be elevated for all emergency department patients,' ... [said] Thomas E. Burroughs, Ph.D., associate professor at St. Louis University Center for Outcomes Research."§

"Many studies have confirmed that the major cause of malpractice claims in EDs [emergency departments] is a failure to diagnose ... As a specialty, EPs [emergency physicians] have developed skills that open them to potential errors in cognition [reasoning] such as confirmation bias ... Put simply, this means that ... [a doctor] may have an initial or a preconceived idea about something and interpret subsequent information or data so as to confirm that idea."**

Just recognize that emergency room doctors, just like others, can make mistakes; and if you've been given a diagnosis, but it doesn't seem right, or you're getting worse, then get another opinion.

*Daudelin, Denise H., and Harry P. Selker. "Medical Error Prevention in ED Triage for ACS: Use of Cardiac Care Decision Support and Quality Improvement Feedback." *Cardiology Clinics* 23 (2005): 601-614, *italics added.*

†Kachalia, Allen, Tejal K. Gandhi, and Ann Louise Puopolo et al. "Missed and Delayed Diagnoses in the Emergency Department: A Study of Closed Malpractice Claims from 4 Liability Insurers." *Annals of Emergency Medicine* 49(2) (2007): 196-205, *italics added.*

‡Holohan, Thomas V., Janice Colestro, John Grippi, Jane Converse, and Michael Hughes. "Analysis of Diagnostic Error in Paid Malpractice Claims with Substandard Care in a Large Healthcare System." *Southern Medical Journal* 98(11) (2005): 1083-1087.

§ED Management. "Most ED Patients Feel Safe, But Many Fear Errors." *ED Management* 17(3) (2005): 33-34.

**Pines, Jesse M. "Profiles in Patient Safety: Confirmation Bias in Emergency Medicine." *Academic Emergency Medicine* 13 (2006): 90-94.

Always trust your intuition

• *You* care the most and know your loved one the best. Listen to your intuition and follow it.

Don't be talked out of it—it could save your loved one's life someday.

Don't stop here. Be sure to read Appendices A and B.

And you really won't understand the book completely until you read the Endnotes.

Appendix A – Why you need a personal health record *now*!

Doctors in practice today only have time to deal with what you've come in for *today*. They don't have time to organize your chart in the ideal fashion, so that they can check to see what tests you need for your chronic condition, or what blood tests to order so that your medication is taken safely, or what preventive measures you need to maintain good health.

And don't think for a moment, "Well, the doctor has everything about me in my chart. I gave him the medical records from the other doctor I was seeing, and he has the lab tests, x-ray reports, and everything for the last ten years."

Here's the problem—he has everything, but no time to organize it. It's just a pile of papers. *You* need to take the initiative to organize your records. And all that you need to do it well is *what you remember about you*. And from here forward, ask your doctor for a copy of each new lab or x-ray report, so that *you* can enter it into your record.

I recommend that you organize your medical information using the PatientFirst Health Record (PFHR), which you can access on the Internet at www.pfhr.org.

For those who worry about putting records on the Internet, the PatientFirst Health Record has the same security as most bank websites. And if you have "I can't sleep" worries about certain facts of your medical information being "out there," then don't put down *that* information. But put the rest of your information there, and then remember to tell the doctor in person of any information you might have excluded.

You don't have to use your social security number, or put down your address, telephone number, or anything that will identify you. And you have total control of it, and can add to it, change it, or delete it at any time.

If you're worried about putting *any* information on the Internet, then put your name down as Bugs Bunny or whomever—just get it done so your medical information is well-organized so that you can help avoid major medical harm. (And try not to be too paranoid—the financial world has already put almost everything about you in major and minor detail where it can be accessed electronically. And this is no different, just much more life-saving.)

So be a good patient—do it for your doctors. It will be such a relief for them to be able to view an encapsulated, organized medical history on you. But you're the one who'll reap the major rewards.

And update it every time you come home from the doctor's office.

Don't put this off! Do it *right now*. There will be no better time.

If you've already decided to make a personal health record for yourself and your loved ones *now*, then go directly to Appendix B. Otherwise, these words are for you:

It's just human nature to say "okay, I can see that's a good idea, and I'll do it as soon as I get around to it." But trust me, *that's not good enough*. For yourself, and for your loved ones, *do it now*. And then print it out, and take the copy to your next doctor's visit of any kind. You'll just need to fill in your medical info as if you were right now in the emergency room or new doctor's office, and you're filling out that form on that clipboard that we all know so well, where you have to answer "what medications are you on," and "what are you allergic to," and "what diseases have you had," and "what operations have you had," etc. But once you do it on the personal health record, you shouldn't ever have to fill out that clipboard form again.

And if you're still tempted to do it *later* for yourself, or maybe your elderly mom or dad, just think about this: if you think it might take up too much of your time now (probably 20-30 minutes, just like those paper ones on a clipboard), think about your doctors, and imagine if they have the time to keep your chart well-organized. The answer to that would be *no*. They no longer have the time. *You're* the one who is harmed if you don't get proper healthcare, and you have more time and personal incentive than the doctor to keep *your* record complete and organized.

So take 20-30 minutes. And do it now. And for your spouse. And for your mother and father, sisters and brothers. (And it also can be used for children, as a place to put their immunizations, and a place to record their doctor visits.)

And if you *still* haven't gone to the computer to do your personal health record–

The Institute of Medicine's Committee on the Quality of Health Care in America believes that you must step forward and participate more in order to get safe and effective healthcare:

"The 21st-century health care system envisioned by the committee—providing care that is evidence-based, patient-centered, and systems-oriented—also implies *new roles and responsibilities for patients and their families, who must become more aware, more participative, and more demanding* in a care system that should be meeting their needs."[A1]

Okay, for those who need one more push–

How bad would you feel if something happened to you or yours, knowing that if you had had the records organized and in a doctor-friendly format, that you could have helped prevent it? And the studies show over and over again that this might be the case. So just like any safety measure you take in your life–like seat belts, pap smears, and mammograms–do it now.

And the reason I've pushed so hard–

I've seen some people who see the technology and say "yeah, that's neat. I'll do it someday."

I just don't want that to be you.

The following quotes describe the importance of having a personal health record:

"*Personal health records* are the information people need to have about their health status and care to understand how they are progressing and to give their history to a new provider. It includes information on their health care providers, current and past medical problems, procedures, current and past medications, allergies, and key test results."[A2]

"*Neglecting the past medical history* can cause a physician inadvertently to discontinue important medications, prescribe an incorrect dose of chronic medications, duplicate a low-yield diagnostic test, neglect an earlier directive or disrupt plans made by previous clinicians."[A3]

"Physician groups, hospitals, and other health care organizations operate as silos, often providing care *without the benefit of complete information* about the patient's condition, medical history, services provided in other settings, or medications prescribed by other clinicians."[A1]

"Effective methods of communication, both among caregivers and between caregivers and patients, are critical to providing high-quality care. *Personal health information* must accompany patients as they transition from home to clinical office setting to hospital to nursing home and back."[A1]

"Medical history and physical examination may lead to misdiagnosis if poorly performed, wrongly interpreted, or only partially conducted. Follow-up diagnostic steps, *such as failure to update medical histories and physical examinations or screen charts in detail, may be neglected.*"[A4]

"When patients see multiple providers in different settings, *none of whom have access to complete information*, it is easier for something to go wrong than when care is better coordinated."[A5]

"*Missing clinical information* has been implicated in injurious adverse events ... Such harm could include otherwise avoidable drug interactions or duplications, missed or delayed diagnoses, missed immunizations, unnecessary testing and procedures, and the downstream effects of such events ... Other studies have demonstrated that errors related to missing clinical information are common and can adversely affect patients."[A6]

A1. Institute of Medicine. *Crossing the Quality Chasm: A New Health System for the 21st Century*. Washington, D.C.: National Academy Press, 2001, pp. 4, 9, 20, *italics added*.

A2. Stead, William W. "Rethinking Electronic Health Records to Better Achieve Quality and Safety Goals." *Annual Review of Medicine* 58 (2007): 35-47, *italics added.*

A3. Redelmeier, Donald A., Jack V. Tu, Michael J. Schull, Lorraine E. Ferris, and Janet E. Hux. "Problems for Clinical Judgment: 2. Obtaining a Reliable Past Medical History." *Canadian Medical Association Journal* 164(6) (2001): 809-813, *italics added.*

A4. Kirch, Wilhelm, and Christine Schafii. "Misdiagnosis at a University Hospital in 4 Medical Eras: Report on 400 Cases." *Medicine* 75(1) (1996): 29-40, *italics added.*

A5. Institute of Medicine. T*o Err Is Human: Building a Safer Health System*. Linda T. Kohn, Janet M. Corrigan, and Molla S. Donaldson, eds. Washington, D.C.: National Academy Press, 2000, p. 3, *italics added.*

A6. Smith, Peter C., Rodrigo Araya-Guerra, and Caroline Bublitz et al. "Missing Clinical Information During Primary Care Visits." *Journal of the American Medical Association* 293(5) (2005): 565-571, *italics added.*

Appendix B – Get started: your personal health record

I recommend the PatientFirst Health Record (PFHR), on the Internet at www.pfhr.org.* It's free, run by a non-profit medical organization, and nobody (other than each patient) accesses the database except for computer maintenance.

(This was the first major effort of my not-for-profit healthcare organization, Patient Always First, because the use of a really great, organized, doctor-friendly personal health record will help you get the best healthcare, and it will also be a great service to your doctors.)

Doctors use a certain format to organize medical records, and the PFHR uses that same format, so that doctors know right where to go to get certain information. *This is critical.* If you just type up whatever, or use a place on the Internet to just "store" medical information that you've typed up—if it's not in a doctor-friendly format—then doctors probably won't even look at it because it's not in the form that's helpful to them. Having an organized and complete record to look at saves a lot of time for doctors, and that saved time could go into having more time for your diagnosis and treatment. Having a *complete, organized* record is very rare in our healthcare system today, and yet it's vital for your health.

It is *very* easy to enter your medical information into this format—it's mostly point-and-click technology, so if you can do anything at all on the computer, you'll be able to do this.

The PFHR has the same online security protection as most bank websites.

Go to www.pfhr.org, and start today to put your information in a doctor-friendly, and patient-empowered form. Pick a username and password, then go directly to the Medication tab, and fill in your medications. Then go to the Diagnoses tab and fill in your history of disease. You can fill out the other tabs later, if you just want to spend a couple of minutes on it now.

One of the really neat things is on the Medications tab. It's really easy to delete a medication, or change a dosage or whatever, and then use the print command, and *voila!* you have a new, neat, printed list of your meds, dosages, and how to take them—not a scrawled list where you've crossed out things, added others, etc.

And all you need to do a good job on this is what *you* remember about *you*! (You don't need to start with your medical records—just like those forms on clipboards, you are just putting down what you remember about yourself.)

Since it's an online record, you can access it from anywhere in the world by going on the Internet to the www.pfhr.org website and putting in your username and password. You'll never be without your medical information ever again!

If you have a group of people that wants to get started, we may even be able to assign one of our directors to walk you through it with video conferencing or speaker phone. Maybe you'd like to organize something like this for your church or social group. All you would need is a computer area, like at a library or school, *or* laptop computers for everyone with hook-ups to the Internet.

On the website, you'll see how to contact us if we can do anything to help you.

The only objection I've seen from doctors is "how do I know what the patient has entered is the truth? How can I rely on that information?" This is so funny, because when you fill out that form on the clipboard, or tell them something in response to their questions, they don't question your truthfulness; but when you have something printed from the computer at home, where you have more time and can be more thorough, then they somehow see it as less trustworthy. So, you might bring this book and let them read this paragraph to realize how illogical that is. *And* tell them that you will vouch for the accuracy of your personal health record by signing it, and they can keep a copy. *You're* the one who will get better medical care because your doctor has a complete, organized history about you, instead of that pile of papers in your chart that he never has time to go through.

An EMT's advice is to put your elderly parent's personal health record on the refrigerator. He says that's where EMTs often look when they come in an emergency. Also, think about having a folder with each family member's latest print-out, so that you can grab it before an emergency trip to the hospital.

So, feel empowered by your decision to take this crucial step to have *organized, doctor-friendly* medical records. Keep them updated when you come home from each doctor's appointment. (There's a "Short-Term Illnesses & Office Visits" subcategory on the History tab.)

Don't believe that your doctor has got it all organized—he doesn't have the time, and you're really more interested in your ongoing health than he is, after all. He's doing the best he can, but ...

---

*There are many options for personal health records on the Internet now—probably close to 200 options. Many are not in the form of medical records that doctors like to use—don't use those. And then most of them have some sort of personal incentive/ulterior motive for you to use *their* record: they want to charge you a yearly fee; they want to make *their* website have the most "hits" so that they can make money from selling advertising; or they want to offer a personal health record to increase the visibility of their commercial organization.

The PatientFirst Health Record is offered to everyone at no charge by a medical non-profit organization, and is only interested in being there for you. It was made with input from patients, computer techs *and* doctors, so it was designed not only to be easy enough for patients to use, but also in the right format and containing the right information that doctors think is valuable.

If you decide to not use the PatientFirst Health Record, just be sure that the personal health record that you choose has all of the features mentioned that make it valuable to you and your doctor.

<u>Easiest steps to start a personal health record</u>

1. Go to www.pfhr.org and click on "Sign up now!"
2. Enter your name and date of birth.
3. Click the "Continue" or "Save Changes" buttons on pages 1, 2 and 3.

4. Choose a username and password on page 4, and choose answers to the security questions so that only *you* can retrieve your password. Click on "Save Changes."

<u>Easiest steps to *use* your personal health record</u>

1. Go to www.pfhr.org and type in your username and password.
2. Click on any of the yellow/gold tabs (like Medications or Diagnoses), then click on the "Add" or "Edit" button in gold on the right side of the page.
3. Enter the information.
4. Click on the "Save Changes" button at the bottom of the page.

Done!

(Click on "Print-Out Options" near the top right of the page to print your record.)

Appendix C – A cool story about how the personal health record has been used

The administrative director of Patient Always First has an 88-year-old father who lives in another state. After a lengthy hospital stay about a year and a half ago, he returned to his home but was no longer able to live alone. Different aides come in to help him as well as a physical therapist who comes to see and work with him twice a week.

Before Betsy used the PFHR, she would ask her dad "are you taking your medicines?" and he would always say "yes." His aide would also say "yes, I give him what he needs."

She decided to start a PFHR for him. She called his pharmacist and got a list of his medicines, and then she called her father's doctor, and asked if these medicines were the ones he should be taking. (She faxed the list to the doctor's office.)

(Doctors would be glad to check a list of medicines like this, because, obviously, they want you on the medicines that they want you on.)

So imagine her surprise when she learned that her father was still taking several medicines that the doctor had discontinued and *replaced* with different prescriptions. The doctor had no way of knowing that his patient was still taking the old medications as well as the new ones. (A real-life scenario of "Medications: just plain mix-ups.") The pharmacy continued to fill all the re-ordered prescriptions, old and new, and because so many different people were coming to the house to help, the aides weren't exactly sure what he was supposed to be taking. The doctor was able to recognize the errors and cross out the medications that were no longer to be given.

Betsy then put her dad's correct medications into the PFHR, and added his diagnoses, allergies, important contacts, etc. as she remembered them and as she asked him to recall. She printed out a copy of the PFHR and it sits on top of the medicine box so that anyone coming in to help can just look at the list and know what medicines to give.

(Remember, *just do it*. From your memory, it's going to be better than what you doctor has had time to organize.)

Then, since the PFHR has this really neat feature where you can let other people access the record, or add to it (only with your permission), she allowed the physical therapist who visits her dad to have access to add to the record. So now, when the physical therapist comes, he types the date, vital signs, and other information about her dad's treatment and condition that day into the record. *And Betsy can see all that information when she logs on.*

So Betsy can have some peace about helping her father long-distance like this—she really is checking in and helping him with his health.

And if her dad should need to go to the emergency room again, then his aide could bring the printed-out PFHR, or Betsy could fax it to the ER, or the ER could even access it online themselves (if Betsy or her father gives them the username and password).

Now, how cool is that?

Don't stop yet. You really won't understand the book completely until you read the Endnotes.

Endnotes

Endnote 1

Medical Errors and Patient Safety

"In 2000, the Institute of Medicine [IOM] issued a landmark report announcing that up to 100,000 Americans die annually due to medical errors. The findings of the Institute of Medicine drew attention to a growing body of research showing that modern health care delivery poses significant patient safety risks, ranging from medication errors to surgical mistakes and from missed diagnoses to treatment delays."[1a]

That makes medical errors in hospitals the 6th leading cause of death—more than those lost through breast cancer, AIDS, or even car accidents.[1b] In fact, the deaths from those three killers *added together* comes to about 99,000 lives per year.[1c] The Institute of Medicine continues:

"Tens of thousands of Americans die each year from errors in their care, and hundreds of thousands suffer or barely escape from nonfatal injuries."[1d]

"That can't be true," you might say. "If that were true, that would be *huge*. We would all know about it, and there would be legislation, fund-raising, marathons, and telethons to fight this major killer. We would all know what each of us can do to avoid these unnecessary, prevalent and devastating *errors in medical care*. I mean, we've all been told not to drive drunk, to fasten our seatbelts, to get mammograms, to practice safe sex. So if those statistics were true, certainly we would have all been told what to do to avoid a medical error death. And I'm sure the American healthcare system is pulling together to get a handle on the problem and bring those numbers down."

But you would be wrong. Many have seen the problem and *are* trying to do something to help, and that effort is called "patient safety." But the American healthcare system is so decentralized and disorganized that most *doctors* don't even know about these studies and these statistics, and have never even heard of "patient safety."

"The decentralized and fragmented nature of the health care delivery system (some would say 'nonsystem') also contributes to unsafe conditions for patients, and serves as an impediment to efforts to improve safety."[1b]

And when most doctors don't see the problem—and patients aren't participating in their healthcare—the drive toward better healthcare can only move at a snail's pace.

"Patient safety 'improved slightly' from 2000 to 2005. The fifth annual National Healthcare Quality Report states that patient safety improved at an annual median rate of 1% for 25 measures."[1e]

"Strategies to reduce error and increase patient safety have not been developed or embraced widely by physicians."[1f]

"A 1999 report by the prestigious Institute of Medicine made clear what doctors have long known: Hospitals can be dangerous. ... But after five years and lots of activity, even the most optimistic observer would say that health care is not much safer than it was in 1999."[1g]

And, although the studies cited by the IOM in 2000 reported a medical error rate of 2.9% to 3.7% in the hospitalized patients they studied, a more recent study of 556,899 patients in Wisconsin hospitals found a 13.3% medical injury rate.[1h]

"One in three respondents [to a recent study] reported that they or a family member had experienced a medical error at some point in their life; one fifth of all respondents said it had caused serious health consequences such as death, long-term disability, or pain."[1i]

The good news is that the information in this book will help you get safe care more of the time—that's the intention of the book. The bad news is that, if more Americans don't get involved in this movement, our families, friends, and neighbors will continue to die and have serious injuries at these alarming rates.

1a. Apker, Julie, Larry A. Mallak, and Scott C. Gibson. "Communicating in the 'Gray Zone': Perceptions about Emergency Physician-Hospitalist Handoffs and Patient Safety. *Academic Emergency Medicine* 14 (2007): 884-894, *citing* Institute of Medicine. *To Err Is Human: Building a Safer Health System.* Linda T. Kohn, Janet M. Corrigan, and Molla S. Donaldson, eds. Washington, D.C.: National Academy Press, 2000.

1b. Institute of Medicine. *To Err Is Human: Building a Safer Health System.* Linda T. Kohn, Janet M. Corrigan, and Molla S. Donaldson, eds. Washington, D.C.: National Academy Press, 2000, p. 3.

1c. Centers for Disease Control and Prevention, www.cdc.gov/nchs/fastats, *accessed* July 31, 2008.

1d. Institute of Medicine. *Crossing the Quality Chasm: A New Health System for the 21st Century*. Washington, D.C.: National Academy Press, 2001, p. 2.

1e. Thompson, Cheryl A. "Government Says Patient Safety Improved 1% Annually for 2000-05." *American Journal of Health-System Pharmacy* 65 (2008): 692-693.

1f. Awad, Samir S., Shawn P. Fagan, and Charles Bellows et al. "Bridging the Communication Gap in the Operating Room with Medical Team Training." *American Journal of Surgery* 190 (2005): 770-774.

1g. Wachter, Robert M., and Kaveh G. Shojania. *Internal Bleeding*. New York City, New York: Rugged Land, 2004, p. 20.

1h. Guse, Clare E., Hongyan Yang, and Peter M. Layde. "Identifying Risk Factors for Medical Injury." *International Journal for Quality in Health Care* 18(3) (2006): 203-210.

1i. Clancy, Carolyn M., Mary Beth Farquhar, and Beth A. Collins Sharp. "Patient Safety in Nursing Practice." *Journal of Nursing Care Quality* 20(3) (2005): 193-197.

More Information about Patient Safety on the Internet

Here are other sources to learn more about patient safety:

▪ The **Agency for Healthcare Research and Quality**, at www.ahrq.gov, is an organization that has made great strides in patient safety in the last few years. It is part of the United States Department of Health and Human Services. Type "patient safety" into the search box at that website. You'll find guidance about preventing medical errors and becoming more involved in your healthcare.

Of note. the U.S. allocates much less funding to promote quality healthcare and prevent medical errors than other developed countries do. And this lack of investment in the quality of our healthcare shows. We are ranked 37th in the world on quality by the World Health Organization,* "last place among [industrialized] countries in preventing deaths through use of timely and effective medical care,"† "last in preventable mortality, just below Ireland and Portugal,"† and "in the lowest 25% of industrialized countries when it comes to infant mortality and life expectancy."*

We need to step up and fund this effort seriously.

*Mestel, Rosie. "Despite Big Spending, U.S. Ranks 37th in Study of Global Health Care." *Los Angeles Times*, June 21, 2000, *citing a report by the World Health Organization*.

†Abelson, Reed. "While the U.S. Spends Heavily on Health Care, a Study Faults the Quality." *New York Times*, July 17, 2008, *citing a report by the Commonwealth Fund*.

▪ The **Institute for Healthcare Improvement**, found at www.ihi.org, is another important patient safety organization. It plans, develops, offers and encourages strategies that hospitals can use to make patient care safer and better. It has been able to make a big dent in decreasing medical errors, saving lives, and improving the quality of care that hospitalized patients have received in the last several years.

▪ The **Joint Commission**, at www.jointcommission.org, is an organization that accredits hospitals and other healthcare facilities, and along the way, facilitates reform by insisting that hospitals implement many programs that increase the safety and quality of patient care. Type "patient safety" into the search box at that website.

Extremely impressive is its recent "Speak Up Initiative." See at www.jointcommission.org/PatientSafety/SpeakUp.

▪ The **National Patient Safety Foundation** website is www.npsf.org. This organization was created in 1995 by the American Medical Association. It makes resources available that "include numerous fact sheets about patient safety with links to other organizations that are involved in the patient-safety agenda. One resource produced by the NPSF ... is titled Nothing About Me, Without Me. This document is a call to all health care organizations to involve patients and their family members in safety initiatives."*

*Beyea, Suzanne C. "Encouraging Patients to Participate in Their Health Care." *AORN Journal* 85(6) (2007): 1231-1233.

You can also Google "patient safety" and find a plethora of other sites that deal with patient safety issues.

More Quotes and Statistics

If you want to read more quotes and statistics on patient safety and medical errors, see below:

"The figures used in the IOM [Institute of Medicine] report probably underestimate the extent of preventable medical injuries because they are based on data extracted from medical records and pertain only to hospitalized patients. Many injuries are not recorded in medical records, either deliberately or as a result of inattention, or because they are not recognized."

Richardson, William C., Donald M. Berwick, and J. Cris Bisgard. Correspondence: "The Institute of Medicine Report on Medical Errors." *New England Journal of Medicine* 343(9) (2000): 663-665.

"The actual numbers range from the IOM's 2000 account of 98,000 deaths per year to HealthGrades 195,000 deaths in each of the years 2000, 2001 and 2002 due to potentially preventable medical errors. Then there's a well-documented hunch by the Agency for Healthcare Research and Quality we may have lost an additional 490,000 patients between 2001 and 2004 due to our failure to improve patient safety."

Hardy, Jeff. "No Hidden Patient: A Safety Design Model." *Trustee* 2007 (February): 32-33.

"An average of 195,000 people in the U.S. died due to potentially preventable, in-hospital medical errors in each of the years 2000, 2001 and 2002, according to a new study of 37 million patient records that was released today by HealthGrades, the healthcare quality company ... 'The equivalent of 390 jumbo jets full of people are dying each year due to likely preventable, in-hospital medical errors,'" said HealthGrades' vice president of medical affairs.

HealthGrades. www.healthgrades.com/media/DMS/pdf/InhospitalDeathsPatientSafety PressRelease072704.pdf, *accessed* July 24, 2008.

"Yet silence surrounds this issue [medical errors]. For the most part, consumers believe they are protected. Media coverage has been limited to reporting of anecdotal cases."

Institute of Medicine. *To Err Is Human: Building a Safer Health System.* Linda T. Kohn, Janet M. Corrigan, and Molla S. Donaldson, eds. Washington, D.C.: National Academy Press, 2000, p. 3.

"We found about thirty publications published during the last ten to twelve years substantiating serious and widespread errors in health care delivery that resulted in frequent avoidable injuries to patients."

Institute of Medicine. *Crossing the Quality Chasm: A New Health System for the 21st Century*. Washington, D.C.: National Academy Press, 2001, pp. 24-25.

"The goal of this report is to break this cycle of inaction. The status quo is not acceptable and cannot be tolerated any longer ... It is simply not acceptable for patients to be harmed by the same health care system that is supposed to offer healing and comfort."

Institute of Medicine. *To Err Is Human: Building a Safer Health System.* Linda T. Kohn, Janet M. Corrigan, and Molla S. Donaldson, eds. Washington, D.C.: National Academy Press, 2000, p. 3.

"A significant percentage of health care consumers continue to believe that the quality of their health care has declined since IOM's report was disseminated, and they are concerned about the care that their families may receive. It seems their concerns may be valid, given the results of The Leapfrog Group's hospital survey. Incredibly, 70% of hospitals surveyed did not have protocols to ensure adequate nursing staff and no policy to ensure that patients understand procedure risks, 60% did not have procedures for preventing malnutrition in patients, 50% did not have procedures in place to prevent bed sores, and 40% did not have handwashing policies that require workers to wash their hands before and after seeing a patient ... If we know better, why are we not doing better?"

Roberts, Velma, and Martha M. Perryman. "Creating a Culture for Health Care Quality and Safety." *The Health Care Manager* 26(2) (2007): 155-158, *citing* Leapfrog Group, www.leapfroggroup.org, *accessed* June 6, 2006.

"Errors in the health care industry are at an unacceptably high level."

Institute of Medicine. *To Err Is Human: Building a Safer Health System.* Linda T. Kohn, Janet M. Corrigan, and Molla S. Donaldson, eds. Washington, D.C.: National Academy Press, 2000, p. 69.

"If truth be told, nobody really knows the extent of medical errors in the practice of health care. Various estimates have put the number of deaths due to medical errors in the United States at 50,000 to 100,000 patients per year or, more graphically, as many as a jumbo jet full of people crashing each and every day ... While authorities may quibble over the details, there is no doubt that medical errors are a major problem within our healthcare system."

Murphy, Joseph G., and William Dunn. Editorial: "Transparency in Health Care: An Issue Throughout U.S. History." *Chest* 133(1) (2008).

"Although the risk of dying as a result of a medical error far surpasses the risk of dying in an airline accident, a good deal more public attention has been focused on improving safety in the airline industry than in the health care industry."

Institute of Medicine. *To Err Is Human: Building a Safer Health System.* Linda T. Kohn, Janet M. Corrigan, and Molla S. Donaldson, eds. Washington, D.C.: National Academy Press, 2000, p. 42.

"The application of engineering concepts to the design of care processes is a critical first step in improving patient safety. Yet few health care organizations have applied the lessons learned by other high-risk industries that have led to very low rates of injury ... Although many, often simple, steps could be taken now and without great cost, knowledge about such actions has neither been disseminated among health care institutions nor widely implemented, probably because *there are often no real penalties for failing to do so* and no real rewards for effective improvements."

Institute of Medicine. *Crossing the Quality Chasm: A New Health System for the 21st Century*. Washington, D.C.: National Academy Press, 2001, pp. 29-30, *italics added.*

"Errors in health care are a leading cause of death and injury. Yet, the American public is seemingly unaware of the problem, and the issue is not getting the attention it should from leaders in the health care industry and the professions. Additionally, the knowledge that has been used in other industries to improve safety [aviation, e.g.] is rarely applied in health care."

Institute of Medicine. *To Err Is Human: Building a Safer Health System.* Linda T. Kohn, Janet M. Corrigan, and Molla S. Donaldson, eds. Washington, D.C.: National Academy Press, 2000, p. 70.

"Hospitals and physicians are paid the same regardless of the safety of the care they deliver. The system thus creates no incentive to invest in safety."

Wachter, Robert M. "The End of the Beginning: Patient Safety Five Years after 'To Err Is Human.'" *Health Affairs* July-December (2004) (Suppl. Web Exclusives): W4-534 – W4-545.

"Health care is not as safe as it should be. A substantial body of evidence points to medical errors as a leading cause of death and injury."

Institute of Medicine. *To Err Is Human: Building a Safer Health System.* Linda T. Kohn, Janet M. Corrigan, and Molla S. Donaldson, eds. Washington, D.C.: National Academy Press, 2000, p. 26.

"In sum, health care is plagued today by a serious quality gap."

Institute of Medicine. *Crossing the Quality Chasm: A New Health System for the 21st Century*. Washington, D.C.: National Academy Press, 2001, p. 35.

Endnote 2

Medical Errors and the Media

"Major accidents, such as Three Mile Island or the *Challenger* accident grab people's attention and make the front page of newspapers. Because they usually affect only one individual at a time, *accidents in health care delivery are less visible and dramatic* than those in other industries. Except for celebrated cases ... they are rarely noticed."[2a]

"In most other industries, when an accident occurs the worker and the company are directly affected. There is a saying that the pilot is always the first at the scene of an airline accident. In health care, the damage happens to a third party; the patient is harmed; the health professional or the organization, only rarely. Furthermore, harm occurs to only one patient at a time; not whole groups of patients, making the accident less visible."[2a]

"Errors occur in all industries ... In health care, events are well publicized [only] when they appear to be particularly egregious—for example, wrong-site surgery or the death of a patient during what is thought to be a routine, low-risk procedure. *Generally, however, accidents are not well publicized; indeed, they may not be known even to the patient or to the family.*"[2a]

"The invisibility of injuries to patients makes them seem trivial or infrequent."[2b]

Just think: when almost 100,000 patients die from medical errors in hospitals every year, that would only be (on average) about 3 patients every 2 months for each hospital.[2c] These are sick patients in the hospital who just quietly die—from *preventable* medical events that caused their deaths. But the low numbers and quiet deaths just don't hit the radar screens of most doctors, nurses, hospital administrators, news agencies, or the American public.

2a. Institute of Medicine. *To Err Is Human: Building a Safer Health System.* Linda T. Kohn, Janet M. Corrigan, and Molla S. Donaldson, eds. Washington, D.C.: National Academy Press, 2000, pp. 51, 53, 158, *italics added.*

2b. Berwick, Donald M. Sounding Board: "Errors Today and Errors Tomorrow." *New England Journal of Medicine* 348(25) (2003): 2570-2572.

2c. *See* Berwick, Donald M. Sounding Board: "Errors Today and Errors Tomorrow." *New England Journal of Medicine* 348(25) (2003): 2570-2572.

Endnote 3

Acute and Chronic Disease Management (and Mismanagement)

It's very difficult for doctors to keep up on current nationally recommended medical guidelines to help *your* illness go away or not get worse:

"In the current health care system, scientific knowledge about best care is not applied systematically or expeditiously to clinical practice. An average of *about 17 years* is required for new knowledge generated by randomized controlled trials to be incorporated into practice, and even then application is highly uneven."[3a]

"Today, no one clinician can retain all the information necessary for sound, evidence-based practice. No unaided human being can read, recall, and act effectively on the volume of clinically relevant scientific literature."[3a]

There are recommended national guidelines on the correct way to treat many chronic and acute illnesses. An important 2003 study selected 30 short-term illnesses, chronic illnesses, and preventive care issues and measured how often optimum interventions were prescribed. They found that patients received, on average, only 54.9% of recommended care.

"The deficits we have identified in adherence to recommended processes for basic care pose serious threats to the health of the American public."[3b]

"Overall, participants received *about half* of the recommended processes involved in care."[3b]

Americans are not receiving recommended care by their doctors 45% of the time. Researchers call this "underuse" of healthcare. We also have a problem where doctors are giving medications, procedures and treatments that are *not* recommended. This "overuse" of care, where patients receive care that is not recommended and is potentially harmful, has been found over 11% of the time.[3b]

"Americans should be able to count on receiving care that meets their needs and is based on the best scientific knowledge. Yet there is strong evidence that this frequently is not the case."[3a]

"Patients with chronic conditions, for which certain routine examinations and tests are crucial in order to prevent complications, do not all get the care they need. Diabetes mellitus causes several complications that are less likely to occur with good care."[3a]

"The extreme variability in practice in clinical areas in which there is strong scientific evidence and a high degree of expert consensus about best practices indicates that current dissemination efforts fail to reach many clinicians and patients, and that there are insufficient tools and incentives to promote rapid adoption of best practices."[3a]

"The dominant finding in our review is that there are large gaps between the care people should receive and the care they do receive. This is true for preventive, acute, and chronic care, whether one goes for a checkup, a sore throat, or diabetic care. It is true whether one looks at overuse [when a health care service is provided although the potential risks outweigh the potential benefits], underuse [when a health care service is *not* provided when the potential benefits outweigh the potential risks], or misuse [when otherwise appropriate care is provided in a manner that leads to or could lead to avoidable complications]. It is true in different types of health care facilities and for different types of health insurance. It is true for all age groups, from children to the elderly. And it is true whether one is looking at the whole country or a single city."[3a]

Bodenheimer reported [from other studies] that patients with diabetes don't get the blood tests they need to assess how well their disease is controlled, and don't get the eye exams they need to save their eyesight. He reported that only 14% of patients with heart disease had achieved the lower cholesterol levels recommended by national guidelines for patients with heart disease.[3c]

A study by Canto et al. found that in patients who presented with heart attacks, *less than 60%* (of those who qualified for it) *received the most recommended treatment* (to dissolve or remove the clot to restart the blood flow to the heart muscle). And with an estimated 1 million people in the U.S. having heart attacks every year—this would mean over 400,000 people are not getting the best treatment to save their heart muscle![3d]

"Overall, only 57 percent of the study patients who were eligible to receive reperfusion therapy received such therapy."[3d]

And it doesn't seem to be getting much better, as noted in a 2005 study by Hayward et al. They noted that although preventing injury from medical errors was a very important part of patient safety, the "overwhelming majority" of medical errors "were related to people getting *too little medical care*, especially for those with *chronic medical conditions*."[3e]

3a. Institute of Medicine. *Crossing the Quality Chasm: A New Health System for the 21st Century*. Washington, D.C.: National Academy Press, 2001, pp. 1, 13-14, 236, 237, *italics added*.

3b. McGlynn, Elizabeth A., Steven M. Asch, and John Adams et al. "The Quality of Health Care Delivered to Adults in the United States." *New England Journal of Medicine* 348(26) (2003): 2635-2645, *italics added*.

3c. Bodenheimer, Thomas. "The American Health Care System: The Movement for Improved Quality in Health Care." *New England Journal of Medicine* 340(6) (1999): 488-492.

3d. Canto, John G., Jeroan J. Allison, and Catarina I. Kiefe et al. "Relation of Race and Sex to the Use of Reperfusion Therapy in Medicare Beneficiaries with Acute Myocardial Infarction." *New England Journal of Medicine* 342(15) (2000): 1094-1100.

3e. Hayward, Rodney A., Steven M. Asch, Mary M. Hogan, Timothy P. Hofer, and Eve A. Kerr. "Sins of Omission: Getting Too Little Medical Care May Be the Greatest Threat to Patient Safety." *Journal of General Internal Medicine* 20 (2005): 686-691, *italics added*.

Endnote 4

Misdiagnosed

"Within medicine, there are more than a dozen major disciplines and a variety of further subspecialties. They have evolved to deal with >10,000 specific illnesses, all of which must be diagnosed before patient treatment can begin."[4a]

"Medical diagnoses that are wrong, missed, or delayed make up a large fraction of all medical errors and cause substantial suffering and injury. Compared with other types of medical error, however, diagnostic errors receive little attention—a major factor in perpetuating unacceptable rates of diagnostic error."[4b]

"Missed and delayed diagnoses in the ambulatory [outpatient] setting are an important patient safety problem ... Over the past decade, lawsuits alleging negligent misdiagnoses have become the most prevalent type of claim in the United States."[4c]

When looking at a group of 307 malpractice claims alleging missed or delayed diagnoses, 59% (181 cases) "were judged to involve diagnostic errors that led to adverse outcomes," including death for 30% (55 deaths).[4c]

Breakdowns in the opportunity to get the right diagnosis occurred for the following reasons: (1) failure to order an appropriate diagnostic test; (2) failure to create a proper follow-up plan; (3) failure to obtain an adequate history or to perform an adequate physical examination; and (4) incorrect interpretation of a diagnostic test.[4c]

"The prevalence of missed cancer diagnoses in our sample is consistent with previous recognition of this problem as a major quality concern for ambulatory care [outpatient care]."[4c]

"Lack of adherence to guidelines for cancer screening and test ordering is a well-recognized problem."[4c]

"Most primary care physicians work under considerable time pressure ... They practice in a health care system in which test results are not easily tracked, patients are sometimes poor informants, multiple handoffs exist, and information gaps are the norm."[4c]

Tai et al.'s study of *actual* cause of death (determined by autopsy) versus *diagnosed* cause of death (determined by review of the patient's chart), revealed that 19.8% of the patients had an undiagnosed illness at death, and in 44.4% of those cases, if the correct diagnosis had been made, then it would have changed the patient's treatment.[4d]

"Among the 850,000 individuals dying in U.S. hospitals every year, a major diagnosis remains clinically undetected in at least 8.4% of cases (71,400 deaths). The data also suggest that approximately 34,850 of these patients might have survived to discharge had misdiagnosis not occurred … although this is more speculative."[4e]

The authors of the study quoted just above further concluded that the fatalities from these diagnostic errors may not have been included in the Institute of Medicine's estimates of preventable deaths.[4e]

There are many errors in thinking that cause doctors to misdiagnose illnesses. Among them are the *availability heuristic* (where the likelihood of a diagnosis is judged by how easily examples spring to mind), the *anchoring heuristic* (where only the initial impression is pursued), *framing effects* (where different decisions are made depending on how the information is presented), and *premature closure* (where several alternatives are not pursued).[4f]

"Follow-up may be a feasible strategy to prevent cognitive shortcuts from causing harm, since it allows clinicians to reconsider the entire picture from an alternative perspective … Diligent follow-up is no panacea for mistakes in reasoning, but it allows for corrective intervention for the patient at hand and the opportunity to learn from mistakes for the benefit of future patients. The caveat to follow-up is that it requires appropriate timing because some clinical problems are irreparable if they are delayed too long … Indeed, the general failure to follow up is the root cause that allows cognitive errors to sometimes run amok in human judgment and decision making."[4f]

Misdiagnosis rates have held steady from 1960 through 1996 at rates of about 10%.

"In spite of the growth in diagnostic technology, the rate of misdiagnosis has not decreased during the last 30 years ... The introduction of new diagnostic procedures such as ultrasound, computerized tomography, and radionuclide scans has not reduced the rate of misdiagnoses. Misinterpretation, technical errors, and overreliance on these new procedures occasionally contributed directly to diagnostic errors. By contrast, the patient's medical history and physical examination played an important role in the diagnostic process, leading to a correct final diagnosis in 60%-70% of cases."[4g]

Graber et al. quote George Soros, "Once we realize that imperfect understanding is the human condition, there is no shame in being wrong, only in failing to correct our mistakes." They look at the approximately 10-15% rate of diagnostic error as determined by autopsy studies, and they try to determine the reasons for these inaccuracies. They focus on system-related issues versus issues in the way doctors think. Although the system of healthcare has been found to be the greatest threat to patient safety in general, as far as diagnosis errors were concerned, system-related factors contributed to diagnostic error in 65% of the errors, while cognitive factors (how doctors reason and make decisions) contributed to 74% of the errors. And of the cognitive errors, "premature closure" ("the failure to continue considering reasonable alternatives after an initial diagnosis was reached") was the most common cause.[4h]

"The most common misadventures [causing a malpractice lawsuit involving a child] were diagnostic error (39%) ... The most common diagnoses involved in the lawsuits were meningitis, appendicitis, arm fracture, and testicular torsion ... Cases in which the child died were most often from meningitis or pneumonia."[4i]

4a. Croskerry, Pat, and Geoff Norman. "Overconfidence in Clinical Decision-Making." *American Journal of Medicine* 121(5A) (2008): S24-S29.

4b. Graber, Mark. "Diagnostic Errors in Medicine: A Case of Neglect." *Joint Commission Journal on Quality and Patient Safety* 31(2) (2005): 106-113.

4c. Gandhi, Tejal K., Allen Kachalia, and Eric J. Thomas et al. "Missed and Delayed Diagnoses in the Ambulatory Setting: A Study of Closed Malpractice Claims." *Annals of Internal Medicine* 145(7) (2006): 488-496.

4d. Tai, Dessmon Y. H., H. El-Bilbeisi, Sanjiv Tewari, Edward J. Mascha, Herbert P. Wiedemann, and Alejandro C. Arroliga. "A Study of Consecutive Autopsies in a Medical ICU: A Comparison of Clinical Cause of Death and Autopsy Diagnosis." *Chest* 119 (2001): 530-536.

4e. Shojania, Kaveh G., Elizabeth C. Burton, Kathryn M. McDonald, and Lee Goldman. "Changes in Rates of Autopsy-Detected Diagnostic Errors Over Time: A Systematic Review." *Journal of the American Medical Association* 289(21) (2003): 2849-2856.

4f. Redelmeier, Donald A. "The Cognitive Psychology of Missed Diagnoses." *Annals of Internal Medicine* 142(2) (2005): 115-120.

4g. Kirch, Wilhelm, and Christine Schafii. "Misdiagnosis at a University Hospital in 4 Medical Eras: Report on 400 Cases." *Medicine* 75(1) (1996): 29-40.

4h. Graber, Mark L., Nancy Franklin, and Ruthanna Gordon. "Diagnostic Error in Internal Medicine." *Archives of Internal Medicine* 165 (2005): 1493-1499.

4i. Selbst, Steven M., Marla J. Friedman, and Sabina B. Singh. "Epidemiology and Etiology of Malpractice Lawsuits Involving Children in U.S. Emergency Departments and Urgent Care Centers." *Pediatric Emergency Care* 21(3) (2005): 165-169.

Endnote 5

Do Your Own Research

Read Endnote 4 for factual information on misdiagnosed healthcare.

Read Endnote 3 on inadequate management of chronic and acute health problems.

If you still don't want to do your own research, at least you are aware of your chances of getting bad care.

Use the Internet! No other U.S. population has had such a broad, egalitarian chance to access medical information, and much of it is in patient-friendly formats.

And take heart from the following study that showed that a misdiagnosis is often caused *not* by a rare disease, but because a common disease has presented in a less typical way. So you really could be the person to diagnose your illness, because you could take the time to search and try to see which disease your symptoms seem to follow, even if they're not typical. Your doctor often doesn't have the time or extensive knowledge to know and think of all the different ways that a disease may present itself.

> "It is not usually the rare disease that leads to misdiagnosis but rather the atypical [non-typical] ... course of a common and well-known disease."[5a]

Go to www.CautiousPatient.org for help with your research.

5a. Kirch, Wilhelm, and Christine Schafii. "Misdiagnosis at a University Hospital in 4 Medical Eras: Report on 400 Cases." *Medicine* 75(1) (1996): 29-40.

Endnote 6

Medication Errors

"Medication errors alone, occurring either in or out of the hospital, are estimated to account for over 7,000 deaths annually."[6a]

"Because of the immense variety and complexity of medications now available, it is impossible for nurses or doctors to keep up with all of the information required for safe medication use."[6a]

"The average number of new drugs approved per year has doubled since the early 1980s, from 19 to 38."[6b]

"Although an incidence of 27% [potentially serious drug interactions] seems high, the results are consistent with what is known about the potential for adverse drug events in patients *who have contact with several doctors*."[6c]

"Prescribing errors are relatively common. These include administration of drugs or dosages which are inappropriate for the patient because of contraindications or unnoticed adverse reactions, failure to communicate essential information, and errors in transcribing medical records. Many of these errors could be avoided if communication with patients was improved and they were encouraged to speak up when they notice unexplained changes in their medication. Patients who are given full information about the purpose of medicines and their likely effects, including side effects, are more likely to take them as recommended, leading to better health outcomes ... Failure to inform patients is a major cause of non-compliance with treatment recommendations."[6d]

"Inappropriate prescribing is a major patient safety concern in the aged population ... Potentially harmful drug-drug and drug-disease combinations occur in various degrees in outpatient care in the elderly population."[6e]

"Physicians prescribe potentially inappropriate medications for nearly a quarter of all older people living in the community, placing them at risk of drug adverse effects."[6f]

6a. Institute of Medicine. *To Err Is Human: Building a Safer Health System.* Linda T. Kohn, Janet M. Corrigan, and Molla S. Donaldson, eds. Washington, D.C.: National Academy Press, 2000, pp. 2, 38, 194.

6b. Institute of Medicine. *Crossing the Quality Chasm: A New Health System for the 21st Century*. Washington, D.C.: National Academy Press, 2001, p. 26.

6c. Norton, Peter G., and G. Ross Baker. Editorial: "Patient Safety in Cancer Care: A Time for Action." *Journal of the National Cancer Institute* 99(8) (2007): 579-580, *italics added.*

6d. Vincent, C.A., and A. Coulter. "Patient Safety: What About the Patient? *Quality and Safety in Health Care* 11 (2002): 76-80.

6e. Zhan, Chunliu, Rosaly Correa-de-Araujo, and Arlene S. Bierman et al. "Suboptimal Prescribing in Elderly Outpatients: Potentially Harmful Drug-Drug and Drug-Disease Combinations." *Journal of the American Geriatric Society* 53 (2005): 262-267.

6f. Willcox, Sharon M., David U. Himmelstein, and Steffie Woolhandler. "Inappropriate Drug Prescribing for the Community-Dwelling Elderly." *Journal of the American Medical Association* 272(4) (1994): 292-296. This article also lists 23 medications that the consensus panel agreed should not be given to the elderly, except in very specific and rare occasions.

Endnote 7

After-Hours Telephone Calls

A physician described one disastrous outcome of telephone medicine:

"Two years ago a 41 year-old English journalist died from septicemia. Her case haunts me. Two days before the Easter weekend Penny Campbell had an injection for hemorrhoids. During the weekend she became progressively unwell and called the out-of-hours medical service ***eight times. None of the doctors she contacted realized how ill she was***. By the next day the die was cast; within 24 hours she was dead."[7a]

In 2007 Killip et al. decided to study the safety of after-hours telephone medicine because of the possible dangers.

"Threats to patient safety were suspected for several reasons. Telephone medicine removes visual cues. Clinicians use cues in the office setting, such as general appearance of patients, to decide which patients may be sicker than others. [And] after-hours telephone medicine may be conducted when the doctor is sleepy or distracted and is often without access to patient records. The potential for harm to patients appears to be high."[7b]

They found:

"There are many, sometimes potentially serious, threats to patient safety in telephone medicine."[7b]

And they concluded:

"After-hours telephone medicine is not as safe as many of us have assumed. Our study demonstrated threats to patient safety. It showed that errors are common, and adverse events are possible."[7b]

7a. Richards, Tessa. "Who Is at the Helm on Patient Journeys?" *British Medical Journal* 335 (2007): 76, *italics and bold type added.*

7b. Killip, Shersten, Carol L. Ireson, Margaret M. Love, Steven T. Fleming, Whitney Katirai, and Katherine Sandford. "Patient Safety in After-Hours Telephone Medicine." *Family Medicine* 39(6) (2007): 404-409.

Endnote 8

Reassuring Telephone Advice

Re-read sections "The problem with after-hours phone calls to your out-of-office doctor" and "Phone calls to the doctor when he is in the office." Re-read Endnote 7.

If you call a telephone hotline where a medical person asks specific questions from a protocol written by doctors for that purpose, then the advice that you get will be much safer than if the medical person is just "winging it" on his own. Remember, though, that he's using a book—a manual—just like the person whom you call with a question about why your computer won't "see" your new printer.

But otherwise, you're not on safe ground at all.

Under a section that says "The Telephone: False Reassurance?" Goldman and Kirtane wrote that in a case where a patient with chest pain telephoned triage nurses for advice on what to do (3 times!), "well-meaning triage nurses seem to have relied on the patient's willingness to be reassured rather than insisting that the patient come to the emergency department for immediate evaluation." This patient was subsequently found to have a missed diagnosis of a heart attack.[8a]

8a. Goldman, Lee, and Ajay J. Kirtane. "Triage of Patients with Acute Chest Pain and Possible Cardiac Ischemia: The Elusive Search for Diagnostic Perfection." *Annals of Internal Medicine* 139(12) (2003): 987-995. The authors believe that, given the potential seriousness of chest pain, "triage systems should recommend immediate in-person evaluation ..., preferably in an emergency department."

Endnote 9

Procedures and Operations

"The quality of health care provided in the United States varies among hospitals, cities, and states. Whether the care is preventive, acute, or chronic, it frequently does not meet professional standards ... A large part of our quality problem is the amount of *inappropriate care* [overuse, such as unneeded procedures and operations] provided in this country."[9a]

The following articles were quoted in the "Procedures and operations: studies show a lot of inappropriate use" section of the text:

Bernstein, Steven J., Elizabeth A. McGlynn, and Albert L. Siu et al. "The Appropriateness of Hysterectomy: A Comparison of Care in Seven Health Plans." *Journal of the American Medical Association* 269(18) (1993): 2398-2402.

Bernstein, Steven J., Lee H. Hilborne, and Lucian L. Leape et al. "The Appropriateness of Use of Coronary Angiography in New York State." *Journal of the American Medical Association* 269(6) (1993): 766-769.

Chassin, Mark R., Jacqueline Kosecoff, and Constance M. Winslow et al. "Does Inappropriate Use Explain Geographic Variations in the Use of Health Care Services?: A Study of Three Procedures." *Journal of the American Medical Association* 258(18) (1987): 2533-2537.

Leape, Lucian L., Lee H. Hilborne, and Rolla Edward Park et al. "The Appropriateness of Use of Coronary Artery Bypass Graft Surgery in New York State." *Journal of the American Medical Association* 269(6) (1993): 753-760.

9a. Institute of Medicine. *Crossing the Quality Chasm: A New Health System for the 21st Century*. Washington, D.C.: National Academy Press, 2001, p. 240, *italics added.*

Endnote 10

Stay with Your Hospitalized Loved One

"Errors in intensive care units (ICUs) seem to be occurring with extraordinary frequency, with reported rates as high as 1.7 per patient per day."[10a]

"Between 3% and 16% of patients experience one or more harmful adverse events while hospitalized and about half of these events are preventable."[10b]

"A major unused resource in most hospitals, clinics, and practices is the patient. Not only do patients have a right to know the medications they are receiving, the reasons for them, their expected effects and possible complications, they also should know what the pills or injections look like and how often they are to receive them."[10c]

"Patients in the ICU have been shown to be particularly susceptible to experiencing a medical error."[10d]

"Medication-related errors occur frequently in hospitals ... about two out of every 100 admissions experienced a preventable adverse drug event."[10c]

"Medication errors were common (nearly 1 of every 5 doses in the typical hospital and skilled nursing facility) ... Assuming 10 doses per patient day, this would mean the typical patient was subject to about two errors every day ... [These] error rates are likely to be understated... The Institute of Medicine report[s] that the medication delivery and administration systems of the nation's hospitals and skilled nursing facilities have major system problems."[10e]

"The Joint Commission has launched a national campaign called the Speak Up™ Initiative that is designed to help patients and their families become aware of their rights. The underlying belief is that by asking questions and knowing their rights, patients have a greater chance of receiving proper care. [Among other things], the campaign advises patients that they have the right to ... receive treatment for pain, be informed about the care they should expect, expect that their opinion will be heard, receive an up-to-date list of their current medications, and receive treatment with respect and courtesy ... Involve family and friends in patient care by designating someone to be an advocate to obtain information and ask questions ... Because of the law requiring private patient information, a form should be signed allowing patient information to be shared with the advocate.".[10f]

The Joint Commission's Speak Up Program

"**S**peak up if you have questions or concerns, and if you don't understand, ask again. It's your body and you have a right to know.

Pay attention to the care you are receiving. Make sure you're getting the right treatments and medications by the right health care professionals. Don't assume anything.

Educate yourself about your diagnosis, the medical tests you are undergoing, and your treatment plan.

Ask a trusted family member or friend to be your advocate.

Know what medications you take and why you take them. Medication errors are the most common health care mistakes.

Use a hospital, clinic, surgery center, or other type of health care organization that has undergone a rigorous on-site evaluation against established state-of-the-art quality and safety standards, such as that provided by The Joint Commission.

Participate in all decisions about your treatment. You are the center of the health care team."[10g]

10a. Manojlovich, Milisa, and Barry DeCicco. "Healthy Work Environments, Nurse-Physician Communication, and Patients' Outcomes." *American Journal of Critical Care* 16(6) (2007): 536-543.

10b. Norton, Peter G., and G. Ross Baker. "Patient Safety in Cancer Care: A Time for Action." *Journal of the National Cancer Institute* 99(8) (April 18, 2007): 579-580. *citing* G. R. Baker, P. G. Norton, and V. Flintoft et al. "The Canadian Adverse Events Study: The Incidence of Adverse Events among Hospital Patients in Canada." *Canadian Medical Association Journal* 170 (2004): 1678-1686.

10c. Institute of Medicine. *To Err Is Human: Building a Safer Health System.* Linda T. Kohn, Janet M. Corrigan, and Molla S. Donaldson, eds. Washington, D.C.: National Academy Press, 2000, pp. 2, 196-197, *italics added.*

10d. Reader, Tom W., Rhona Flin and Brian H. Cuthbertson. "Communication Skills and Error in the Intensive Care Unit." *Current Opinion in Critical Care* 13 (2007): 732-736.

10e. Barker, Kenneth N., Elizabeth A. Flynn, Ginette A. Pepper, David W. Bates, and Robert L. Mikeal. "Medication Errors Observed in 36 Health Care Facilities." *Archives of Internal Medicine* 162 (2002): 1897-1903.

10f. Sandlin, Debbie. "The Joint Commission's Speak Up™ Initiative." *Journal of PeriAnesthesia Nursing* 22(6) (2007): 438-439.

10g. The Joint Commission. "Speak Up™ Program: Facts about Speak Up Initiatives." www.jointcommission.org/GeneralPublic/Speak+Up/about_speakup.htm, *accessed* November 15, 2008.

Endnote 11

Nurses and Good Hospital Care

"Registered nurses play a crucial role in protecting patients from harm. Nurses act as a hospital unit's frontline against error ... This analysis investigated the influence of job demands on nurses' perception of patient safety, or the ability to protect their patients from medical errors or complications ... Nurses who have higher demands perceive a decreased ability to provide safe care ... Nurses appear to be aware when organizational demands surpass their ability to protect the patients from injury and medical complications."[11a]

"Nurses constitute the surveillance system for early detection of patient complications and problems, and are in the best position to initiate actions that minimize negative patient outcomes."[11b]

"Units with higher [nurse] staffing had lower incidence of CLBSI [central line associated bloodstream infections], ventilator-associated pneumonia, 30-day mortality, and decubiti [bed sores] ... Nurse working conditions were associated with all outcomes measured. Improving working conditions will most likely promote patient safety."[11c]

"In a survey ... 2%-5% of nurses work more than 60 hours a week, 28% work shifts that are 12 hours or longer, and in intensive care units (ICUs), 36% work more than 12 hours a day ... It has been shown that working these sustained hours can affect the ability to provide safe patient care as well as strain interpersonal relationships, increase stress in the work environment, and contribute to physiological implications."[11d]

"[Nurse] staffing is a key determinant of healthcare-associated infection in critically ill patients. Assuming causality, a substantial proportion of all infections could be avoided if nurse staffing were to be maintained at a higher level."[11e]

"Nurses significantly impact health care ... Studies suggest poor patient outcomes, such as increased infections and respiratory failure, occur when there is inadequate nursing staff. Furthermore, nurses thwart medical errors. For example, nursing staff have been shown to intercept almost 90% of medication errors before they reach patients ... Most disturbing is that over 75% of these nurses [in the survey] reported that unsafe working conditions interfered with the ability to deliver quality care

... Seventy-five percent of the nurses surveyed indicated the quality of nursing care at their facility had deteriorated over the preceding 2 years ... Studies show an association between poor nurse staffing levels and adverse patient outcomes ... [A study by Aiken et al.] found that each additional patient per nurse was associated with a 7% increase in both patient mortality and deaths following complications ... These findings provide significant information regarding our health system and the gap in quality and performance."[11f]

"Among medical patients, a higher proportion of hours of care per day provided by registered nurses and a greater absolute number of hours of care per day provided by registered nurses were associated with a shorter length of stay and lower rates of both urinary tract infections and upper gastrointestinal bleeding. A higher proportion of hours of care provided by registered nurses was also associated with lower rates of pneumonia, shock or cardiac arrest, and "failure to rescue," which was defined as death from pneumonia, shock or cardiac arrest, upper gastrointestinal bleeding, sepsis, or deep venous thrombosis ... As hospitals have responded to financial pressure from Medicare, managed care, and other private payers, registered nurses have become increasingly dissatisfied with the working conditions in hospitals. They report that they are spending less time taking care of increasingly ill patients and believe that the safety and quality of inpatient care are deteriorating."[11g]

"A growing body of research ties nurse staffing to patient outcomes, reinforcing the important role of nursing in the delivery of safe, efficacious health care ... Nurses identify staffing issues as critical to the delivery of optimal patient care."[11h]

"The risks of making an error were significantly increased when work shifts were longer than twelve hours, when nurses worked overtime, or when they worked more than forty hours per week."[11i]

11a. Ramanujam, Rangaraj, Kathleen Abrahamson, and James G. Anderson. "Influence of Workplace Demands on Nurses' Perception of Patient Safety." *Nursing and Health Sciences* 10 (2008): 144-150.

11b. Potter, Patricia, Laurie Wolf, and Stuart Boxerman et al. "An Analysis of Nurses' Cognitive Work: A New Perspective for Understanding Medical Errors." www.ncbi.nlm.nih.gov/books/bv.fcgi?rid=aps.section.124, *accessed* July 31, 2008.

11c. Stone, Patricia W., Cathy Mooney-Kane, and Elaine L. Larson et al. "Nurse Working Conditions and Patient Safety Outcomes." *Medical Care* 45(6) (2007): 571-578.

11d. National Association of Neonatal Nurses. "NANN Position Statement 3043: Neonatal Advanced Practice Nurses Shift Length, Fatigue, and Impact on Patient Safety." *Advances in Neonatal Care* 7(6) (2007): 326-329.

11e. Hugonnet, Stephane, Jean-Claude Chevrolet, and Didier Pittet. "The Effect of Workload on Infection Risk in Critically Ill Patients." *Critical Care Medicine* 35(1) (2007): 76-81.

11f. Lin, Laura, and Bryan A. Liang. "Addressing the Nursing Work Environment to Promote Patient Safety." *Nursing Forum* 42(1) (2007): 20-30, *citing* Aiken, L.H., S.P. Clarke, D.M. Sloane, J. Sochalski, and J.H. Silber. "Hospital Nurse Staffing and Patient Mortality, Nurse Burnout, and Job Dissatisfaction." *Journal of the American Medical Association* 288(16) (2002): 1987-1993.

11g. Needleman, Jack., Peter Buerhaus, Soeren Mattke, Maureen Stewart, and Katya Zelevinsky. "Nurse-Staffing Levels and the Quality of Care in Hospitals." *New England Journal of Medicine* 346(22) (2002): 1715-1722.

11h. Riehle, Annette I., Linda S. Hanold, Sharon L. Sprenger, Jerod M. Loeb, and the Joint Commission. "Specifying and Standardizing Performance Measures for Use at a National Level: Implications for Nursing-Sensitive Care Performance Measures." *Medical Care Research and Review* 64(2)(Suppl.) (2007): 64S-81S.

11i. Rogers, Ann E., Wei-Ting Hwang, Linda D. Scott, Linda H. Aiken, and David F. Dinges. "The Working Hours of Hospital Staff Nurses and Patient Safety." *Health Affairs* 23(4) (2004): 202-212.

Endnote 12

Rapid Response Teams

"The rapid response team is designed to bring critical care to the floor patient's bedside with rapid evaluation and resuscitation. Several studies document reduced rates of cardiac arrest, unanticipated ICU admission, and mortality."[12a]

"One contributing factor to the failure to rescue these patients is the failure to recognize a patient's deteriorating clinical condition."[12a]

"The rapid response team concept has evolved as a means of extending critical care outside of the intensive care unit to intervene early and prevent deterioration to cardiac arrest."[12a]

"Rapid response teams (RRTs) have become one of the most widely implemented patient safety interventions in American hospitals, with nearly 3,000 hospitals committing to the implementation of an RRT."[12b]

"There are a sufficient number of reports of benefit to support a recommendation that hospitals implement and locally assess an RRS [rapid response system]."[12c]

12a. Offner, Patrick J., Joseph Heit, and Robin Roberts. "Implementation of a Rapid Response Team Decreases Cardiac Arrest Outside of the Intensive Care Unit." *Journal of Trauma* 62(5) (2007): 1223 1228.

12b. Ranji, Sumant R., and Kaveh G. Shojania. "Implementing Patient Safety Interventions in Your Hospital: What to Try and What to Avoid." *Medical Clinics of North America* 92 (2008): 275-293.

12c. DeVita, Michael A., Rinaldo Bellomo, and Kenneth Hillman et al. "Findings of the First Consensus Conference on Medical Emergency Teams." *Critical Care Medicine* 34(9) (2006): 2463-2478.

Endnote 13

Unpleasant Doctors

In medical studies, doctors who act out, and their inappropriate behaviors, are described as "disruptive." Harm to a patient stemming from medical management is described as an "adverse event."

"Disruptive physician behavior can lead to patient safety issues. Physicians who are intimidating to nursing staff may result in the nurse fearing to clarify an unclear order with the physician because of the negative behavior that frequently occurs with this physician. The nurse may go ahead and give the medication as it seemed to be ordered, and this may result in an error."[13a]

Of these problem physicians, nurses went on to describe condescending voices, impatience with questions, and "a reluctance or refusal to answer questions or telephone calls," in addition to stronger verbal abuse, threatening body language, and actual physical abuse.[13a]

Rosenstein and O'Daniel's survey of the effects of "disruptive" behavior in hospital working settings found:

"The majority of the comments [of the hospital workers that were surveyed] focused on the negative consequences of intimidation and poor communication ... One of the common themes was the hesitation and reluctance to call certain doctors to question or clarify an order in fear of provoking an antagonistic or hostile response. To quote one representative comment: 'Most nurses are afraid to call Dr. X when they need to, and frequently won't call. Their patient's medical safety is always in jeopardy because of this.'"[13b]

The following are some verbatim responses by hospital workers to the Rosenstein and O'Daniel survey:

▪"'Adverse event related to med error because MD would not listen to RN.'

▪ 'RN did not call MD about change in patient condition because he had a history of being abusive when called. Patient suffered because of this.'
▪ 'Cardiologist upset by phone calls and refused to come in. RN told it was not her job to think, just to follow orders. Rx delayed. MI [heart attack] extended.'
▪ 'Difficult endoscopy. Physician angry, frustrated, abusive to patient and technician. Patient safety compromised.'
▪ 'Communication between OB and delivery RN was hampered because of MD behavior. Resulted in poor outcome in newborn.'
▪ 'MD yelled at RN for calling at night, patient condition not addressed, resulting in a negative patient outcome.'
▪ 'RN called MD multiple times re: deteriorating patient condition. MD upset with RN calling. Patient eventually had to be intubated.'
▪ 'Failure of MD to listen to RN regarding patient's condition. Patient had postop pulmonary embolism.'
▪ 'RNs did not want to call MD after IV ran out. No antibiotic therapy for four days. RN afraid to call MD. Patient expired.'
▪ 'Poor communication postop because of disruptive reputation resulted in delayed treatment, aspiration, and eventual demise.'"[13c]

"Disruptive, intimidating, or abusive behavior may increase the likelihood of errors by leading nurses, residents, or colleagues to avoid the disruptive physician, to hesitate to ask for help or clarification of orders, and to hesitate to make suggestions about patient care."[13d]

"Yelling, insulting others, or a refusal to carry out duties are among the common types of [disruptive physician] behaviors reported. The targets of such behavior are often co-workers with less power than the offending individual ... A consequence of this type of behavior is corruption of teamwork."[13e]

"Although most hospitals have policies concerning unacceptable behavior, these policies are often not enforced, particularly when members of the medical staff are involved."[13f]

"As one respondent observed [in a survey on disruptive doctors], 'Physicians too often feel they are above rules, regulations, behavioral standards and other day-to-day social etiquette, as they feel they are a privileged class.'"[13g]

"While the percentage of individuals who exhibit truly disruptive behaviors is small, its effect can permeate throughout the entire organization."[13b]

"Research in the ICU has shown poor communication between team members to be a common causal factor underlying adverse events."[13h]

"Ninety-four percent of OR [operating room] clinicians said disruptive behavior—including yelling, insults, abusive language and even physical assaults—was linked to an adverse event, medical error, compromise in patient safety, impaired quality and patient mortality."[13i]

"Disruptive behavior occurs frequently on labor and delivery units on the West Coast. This behavior contributed to the nursing shortage, near misses, and adverse occurrences, and was exhibited by a broad range of professionals. The behavior was not always effectively managed by the organization ... The spectrum of this type of behavior includes angry outbursts, rudeness, verbal attacks, physical threats or aggressive physical contact, noncompliance with existing policies, sexual harassment, idiosyncratic, inconsistent, or passive aggressive orders, derogatory comments about the organization, and disruption of smooth function of the healthcare team."[13j]

Patients would be safer if physicians were taught to value communication and teamwork (playing well with others?).

We could learn a few safety tips from the aviation industry:

"Military and civilian aviation has taught senior pilots to respect and listen to junior colleagues, and that copilots and junior officers have the responsibility to communicate clearly their concerns about safety. Superiors have the responsibility to reply to these concerns according to the 'two-challenge rule.' This rule states that if a pilot is clearly challenged twice about an unsafe situation during a flight without a satisfactory reply, the subordinate is empowered to take over the controls."[13k]

In one devastating outcome, an 8-year-old boy died during surgery to get ear tubes. During the operation, the operating nurses "observed the anesthesiologist nodding in his chair, head bobbing, [but] they did not speak to him because they 'were afraid of a confrontation.'" This tragic outcome occurred through a series of errors, but of significance is that this doctor's objectionable behavior had been seen before and tolerated, and the nurses failed to act when they saw this doctor fall asleep because of fear of confrontation, to the tragic detriment of this young patient.[13l]

13a. Wlody, Ginger Schafer. "Nursing Management and Organizational Ethics in the Intensive Care Unit. *Critical Care Medicine* 35(2 Suppl.) (2007): S29-S35.

13b. Rosenstein, Alan H., and Michelle O'Daniel. "Managing Disruptive Physician Behavior: Impact on Staff Relationships and Patient Care." *Neurology* 70 (2008): 1564-1570.

13c. Rosenstein, Alan H., and Michelle O'Daniel. "Disruptive Behavior & Clinical Outcomes: Perceptions of Nurses & Physicians." *American Journal of Nursing* 105(1) (2005): 54-64.

13d. Leape, Lucian L., and John A. Fromson. "Problem Doctors: Is There a System-Level Solution?" *Annals of Internal Medicine* 114(2) (2006): 107-115.

13e. ACOG (The American College of Obstetricians and Gynecologists). ACOG Committee Opinion 366: "Disruptive Behavior." *Obstetrics & Gynecology* 109(5) (2007): 1261-1262.

13f. Barden, Connie, and Claudia Distrito. "Toward a Healthy Work Environment." *Health Progress* 86(6) (2005): 16-20.

13g. Manojlovich, Milisa, and Barry DeCicco. "Healthy Work Environments, Nurse-Physician Communication, and Patients' Outcomes." *American Journal of Critical Care* 16(6) (2007): 536-543.

13h. Reader, Tom W., Rhona Flin, and Brian H. Cuthbertson. "Communication Skills and Error in the Intensive Care Unit." *Current Opinion in Critical Care* 13 (2007): 732-736.

13i. Haugh, Richard. "Stop Yelling at Me." *Hospitals & Health Networks* 80(11) (2006): 14.

13j. Veltman, Larry L. "Disruptive Behavior in Obstetrics: A Hidden Threat to Patient Safety." *American Journal of Obstetrics & Gynecology* 196 (2007): 587.e1-587.e5.

13k. Institute of Medicine. *To Err Is Human: Building a Safer Health System.* Linda T. Kohn, Janet M. Corrigan, and Molla S. Donaldson, eds. Washington, D.C.: National Academy Press, 2000, p. 180.

13l. Helmreich, Robert L. "On Error Management: Lessons from Aviation." *British Medical Journal* 320 (2000): 781 785.

Endnote 14

Hospital-Acquired Infections

According to the Center for Disease Control (CDC), there are 1.7 million cases of hospital-associated infections a year, with 99,000 of those patients dying because of the infection, which makes it "one of the top ten leading causes of death in the United States."[14a]

"A lack of consciousness about the impact of hand hygiene and time pressures, along with organizational issues such as inadequate staffing, combine to create an environment in which an average of only 40% of workers comply with good hand-hygiene practices."[14b]

See the "Hand Hygiene Saves Lives" video by the CDC noting that for hospital paticnts "it is appropriate to ask or remind their healthcare providers to practice hand hygiene."[14c] This means to either wash their hands or use an alcohol-based hand sanitizer.

"WHO [the World Health Organization] estimates that at any point in time more than 1.4 million people around the world have a hospital acquired infection and says that many of these infections can be prevented by good hand hygiene."[14d]

"Healthcare-associated infections (HCAIs) represent a major risk to patient safety and contribute towards suffering, prolongation of hospital stay, cost and mortality. Hand hygiene is the core element to protect patients against HCAIs and colonization with multi-resistant microorganisms. Cleansing hands with alcohol-based hand rub is a simple and undemanding procedure that requires only a few seconds. If hand rub is easily available at each point of care, hand hygiene can also easily be integrated in the natural workflow—even in high-density care settings [like ICUs]. However, most healthcare workers practice hand hygiene less than half as often as they should."[14e]

The authors of the above offer a simple, easy-to-remember concept for healthcare workers–what they call "My Five Moments for Hand Hygiene."

▪ 1. Before patient contact [when they come into the room, *after* touching the door, and *before* touching the patient]
▪ 2. Before aseptic task [*before* working with a surgical wound or an IV site on the patient]
▪ 3. After body fluid exposure [*after* handling a urine bag, e.g.]
▪ 4. After patient contact [*after* last physical contact with the patient at that visit]
▪ 5. After contact with patient surroundings [*after* touching anything else in the room, just before leaving the patient's room][14e]

"It is noteworthy that healthcare workers usually touch an object within the patient zone and not the patient before leaving."[14e]

How to best protect your loved one considering all these rules? Although medical personnel are supposed to follow all of the above, *you* can do a lot of good by being mindful of these two special moments when it's most important that hands are cleansed:

1. **When medical personnel first come into the room, and**
2. **Before they touch a surgical site or an IV site, *if* they have touched anything else in the room after the first cleansing.**

And "medical personnel" includes doctors.

If you're in an intensive care unit where patients don't have individual rooms, then the above rules apply whenever the nurse returns to *your* loved one after attending to any other patient or being anywhere else in the ward.

Additional Specific Handwashing Recommendations[14f]

• Healthcare personnel (nurses, doctors, aides, etc.) are supposed to "perform hand hygiene" in these circumstances:

▪"Before and after having direct contact with patients;
▪ after removing gloves;
▪ before handling an invasive device for patient care, regardless of whether or not gloves are used;

▪ after contact with body fluids or excretions, mucous membranes, non-intact skin, or wound dressings;
▪ if moving from a contaminated body site to a clean body site during patient care;
▪ after contact with inanimate objects (including medical equipment) in the immediate vicinity of the patient;"[14f]
▪ and whenever hands look soiled or have potentially been contaminated, and after using the bathroom.

• Hand hygiene should be performed as follows:

▪"Alcohol handrub: apply a palmful of product and cover all surfaces of the hand; rub together until the hands are dry.
▪ Soap and water: wet the hands first and apply enough soap to cover all surfaces of the hands.
▪ Make sure the hands are dry and towels are not used repeatedly or by multiple people.
▪ Water: health settings are encouraged to ensure that water is available for hand hygiene, but in settings without easy access to water, efforts should be made to make available alcohol-based handrubs as a priority."[14f]

• Gloves should be used as follows:

▪"Gloves do not replace the need for hand cleansing with rubs or soap and water.
▪ Gloves protect staff from blood and body fluids, non-intact skin and mucous membranes.
▪ Remove gloves after caring for a patient. Do not use the same pair of gloves for more than one patient.
▪ Change or remove gloves if moving from a contaminated body site to a clean site on the same patient.
▪ Avoid reuse of gloves."[14f]

"[In a hospital handwashing study], average compliance was 48% … Noncompliance was higher among physicians, nursing assistants, and other health care workers than among nurses and was lowest on weekends. Noncompliance was higher in intensive care than in internal medicine units, during procedures that carry a high risk for contamination, and when intensity of patient care was high … On average, infections complicate 7% to 10% of hospital admissions … Transmission of microorganisms from the hands of health care workers is the main cause of nosocomial [hospital-acquired] infections, and handwashing remains the most important preventive measure. Unfortunately, compliance with handwashing is unacceptably low in most institutions ... Understaffing of hospital wards decreases compliance with isolation precautions and increases risk for nosocomial infections."[14g]

14a. http://www.cdc.gov/ncidod/dhqp/hai.html, *accessed* July 26, 2008.

14b. Murphy-Knoll, Linda. "The Joint Commission's Infection Control National Patient Safety Goal." *Journal of Nursing Care Quality* 22(1) (2007): 8-10.

14c. http://www.cdc.gov/handhygiene/Patient_Admission_Video.html, *accessed* July 26, 2008.

14d. Pandey, Kaushal. News: "WHO Launches List of Nine Solutions to Improve Patients' Safety." *British Medical Journal* 334 (2007):974.

14e. Sax, H., B. Allegranzi, I. Uckay, E. Larson, J. Boyce, and D. Pittet. "'My Five Moments for Hand Hygiene': A User-Centered Design Approach to Understand, Train, Monitor and Report Hand Hygiene." *Journal of Hospital Infection* 67 (2007): 9-21.

14f. Allegranzi, Benedetta, Julie Storr, Gerald Dziekan, Agnes Leotsakos, Liam Donaldson, and Didier Pittet. "The First Global Patient Safety Challenge 'Clean Care is Safer Care': From Launch to Current Progress and Achievements." *Journal of Hospital Infection* 65(S2) (2007): 115-123.

14g. Pittet, Didier, Philippe Mourouga, Thomas V. Perneger, and the Members of the Infection Control Program. "Compliance with Handwashing in a Teaching Hospital." *Annals of Internal Medicine* 130(2) (1999): 126-130.

Medical Care of the Future

Some Thoughts from 1981

It's unfortunate that even though many of our current healthcare problems, with proposed solutions, were recognized by Dr. Weed in 1981, we have still not implemented these solutions so many years later.

"The patient's role in his own behalf should be central to the overall health-care effort. He must work with a copy of his record and with modern tools of communication so that he can help make the necessary choices to deal with his health problems ... We should not rely too heavily on human memory ... The aids used to extend memory and analytic capacities should be reliable and capable of being kept up to date ... Since we know that no one can provide total care to another person over that person's entire lifetime, emphasis must shift from the physician to a coordinated system of care through which the efforts of many kinds and levels of providers and of patients themselves are organized and integrated.

Random audits of medical records [should be used to check for appropriate care] ... Without random audits throughout the careers of all health-care providers, performance can deteriorate, especially when one or two of several choices yield more money, convenience, or satisfaction to the providers. All providers cannot always be expected to put the patient's interest first, any more than all citizens can always be expected to figure income taxes correctly, if they are not aware of an established random auditing process ... Thoughtful physicians will not want to be unchallenged 'brokers of the health care system' when everyone—patients particularly—can thrive within a defined system of health care with corrective feedback loops based on educational principles that can be believed in [*nationally-recommended guidelines?*] and based on powerful new tools [*the personal computer and the Internet?*] that couple the best in current thinking with everyday actions."*

*Weed, Lawrence L. Sounding Board: "Physicians of the Future." *New England Journal of Medicine* 304(15) (1981): 903-907.